CULTURES FOR PERFORMANCE IN HEALTH CARE

STATE OF HEALTH SERIES

Edited by Chris Ham, Professor of Health Policy and Management at the University of Birmingham and Director of the Strategy Unit at the Department of Health.

Current and forthcoming titles

CULTURES FOR PERFORMANCE IN HEALTH CARE

Russell Mannion,
Huw T.O. Davies &
Martin N. Marshall

Open University Press

Open University Press
McGraw-Hill Education
McGraw-Hill House
Shoppenhangers Road
Maidenhead
Berkshire
England
SL6 2QL

email: enquiries@openup.co.uk
world wide web: www.openup.co.uk

and Two Penn Plaza, New York, NY 10121-2289, USA

First published 2005

A catalogue record of this book is available from the British Library

ISBN 0 335 21553 X (pb) 0 335 21554 8 (hb)

Library of Congress Cataloging-in-Publication Data
CIP data applied for

Typeset by RefineCatch Limited, Bungay, Suffolk
Printed in Great Britain by MPG Books Ltd, Bodmin, Cornwall

For Judith, Elizabeth, Catherine M, Catherine G, Thomas, Bryn, Padrig and Sue

CONTENTS

LIST OF FIGURES, TABLES AND BOXES

SERIES EDITOR'S INTRODUCTION

Health services in many developed countries have come under critical scrutiny in recent years. In part this is because of increasing expenditure, much of it funded from public sources, and the pressure this has put on governments seeking to control public spending. Also important has been the perception that resources allocated to health services are not always deployed in an optimal fashion. Thus at a time when the scope for increasing expenditure is extremely limited, there is a need to search for ways of using existing budgets more efficiently. A further concern has been the desire to ensure access to health care of various groups on an equitable basis. In some countries this has been linked to a wish to enhance patient choice and to make service providers more responsive to patients as 'consumers'.

Underlying these specific concerns are a number of more fundamental developments which have a significant bearing on the performance of health services. Three are worth highlighting. First, there are demographic changes, including the ageing population and the decline in the proportion of the population of working age. These changes will both increase the demand for health care and at the same time limit the ability of health services to respond to this demand.

Second, advances in medical science will also give rise to new demands within the health services. These advances cover a range of possibilities, including innovations in surgery, drug therapy, screening and diagnosis. The pace of innovation quickened as the end of the twentieth century approached, with significant implications for the funding and provision of services.

Third, public expectations of health services are rising as those who use services demand higher standards of care. In part, this is stimulated by developments within the health service, including the availability of new technology. More fundamentally, it stems from the emergence of a more educated and informed population, in which people are accustomed to being treated as consumers rather than patients.

Against this background, policy makers in a number of countries are reviewing the future of health services. Those countries which have traditionally relied on a market in health care are making greater use of regulation and planning. Equally, those countries which have traditionally relied on regulation and planning are moving towards a more competitive approach. In no country is there complete satisfaction with existing methods of financing and delivery, and everywhere there is a search for new policy instruments.

The aim of this series is to contribute to debate about the future of health services through an analysis of major issues in health policy. These issues have been chosen because they are both of current interest and of enduring importance. The series is intended to be accessible to students and informed lay readers as well as to specialists working in this field. The aim is to go beyond a textbook approach to health policy analysis and to encourage authors to move debate about their issues forward. In this sense, each book presents a summary of current research and thinking, and an exploration of future policy directions.

Professor Chris Ham
Professor of Health Policy and Management at the University of Birmingham and Director, the Strategy Unit, Department of Health

ABOUT THE AUTHORS

Russell Mannion PhD is Senior Research Fellow in the Centre for Health Economics, University of York and Director of the Masters course in Health Economics at the Nuffield Institute for Health, University of Leeds. Russell's research interests encompass: the economics of health service delivery and organization; performance measurement and management; clinical governance; international health policy reform; and the relationship between organizational culture(s) and health care quality. He has authored several books and over 100 journal articles and scientific papers, as well as providing advice to a range of government agencies and professional bodies including the Department of Health, HM Treasury, the Audit Commission, the Commission for Health Improvement, the Modernisation Agency, the Scottish Executive, the NHS Confederation and the International Society for Quality in Health Care.

Russell has a particular interest in interdisciplinary work and has lectured and/or supervised PhD students in the following departments at the University of York: Economics and Related Studies, Health Sciences, Management Studies and Social Policy. He is the external examiner for a range of undergraduate and postgraduate courses in economics and management at the University of St Andrews and the Doctor of Public Health, at the London School of Hygiene and Tropical Medicine. He has held visiting positions in the Facolta di Economia, Universita di Roma 'Tor Vergatta' and the Instituto Superior de Economia e Gestáo, in Lisbon.

Huw Davies MA (Cantab), MSc, PhD, HonMFPHM is Professor of Health Care Policy and Management at the University of St Andrews, and a former Harkness Fellow in Health Care Policy when he was based at the Institute for Health Policy Studies at the University of California, San Francisco. He is Co-Director of both the Centre for Public Policy & Management (CPPM) and the ESRC-funded Research Unit for Research Utilisation (RURU) in the University of St Andrews, and is Deputy Director of the Service Delivery and Organisation (SDO) Research Funding Programme on secondment to the Department of Health. Huw's research interests are in service delivery, encompassing evidence-based policy and practice, performance measurement and management, accountability, governance and trust. He also has a particular interest in the role of organizational culture in the delivery of high quality services. He has published widely in each of these areas, with over 130 papers appearing in peer-reviewed journals. He is also the author or co-author of several books including: *The Audit Handbook* (Wiley 1993); *Research in Health Care* (Wiley 1996); *What Works? Evidence-based Policy and Practice in Public Services* (Policy Press 2000); *Health Services Research: Avoiding Common Pitfalls* (Quay Books 2001); and *Healthcare Performance and Organisational Culture* (Radcliffe Medical Press 2003).

Martin Marshall BSc, MB BS, MSc, MD, FRCGP is Head of the School of Primary Care, Professor of General Practice at the National Primary Care Research and Development Centre, University of Manchester and a part-time general practitioner in an inner-city practice. Prior to this he was a principal in general practice in Exeter for ten years. His research interests are in the field of policy related quality of care: the development, use and abuse of quality indicators in primary care; the public disclosure of information about performance; patient safety in primary care; and the relationship between organizational culture and quality improvement. He was a Harkness Fellow in Health Care Policy in 1998/99, based at the RAND Corporation, California. He was a member of the GMC/RCGP working group that produced Good Medical Practice for General Practitioners, the basis for revalidation of general practitioners. He is currently a member of the RCGP Research Group and the Manchester Performance Panel. He acts as an expert advisor to the Commission for Health Improvement and their Office for Healthcare Information, the Modernisation Agency, the National Clinical Assessment Authority, the National Patient Safety Agency, the National Patient Safety Research Programme and the National Primary Care Collaborative. He is vice-president of the European Society for Quality Improvement in Family Practice and an advisor to the OECD.

FOREWORD BY AIDAN HALLIGAN AND JAY BEVINGTON

The 800 pound gorilla that impairs performance and stifles change is culture

(Pascale *et al.* 1997)

Every organization is the product of the way its members think and interact. Change the way people think and interact, and you can change the world

(Senge 1985)

Cultural transformation is at the heart of the UK government's reforms of the NHS. Culture is the informal psychological and social aspects of an organization that influence how people think, what they see as important and how they behave and interact at work. This book provides empirical evidence of the influence of organizational culture on the performance of health care organizations.

Mannion, Davies and Marshall conclude that culture matters. Conceptualizing people's day-to-day experiences of work in terms of organizational culture and asking them about 'the way things are done' within their workplace resonates well with NHS staff. Staff are fascinated about their organizations' dominant culture and subcultures, and are keen to explore their unique roles and responsibilities in maintaining or changing those cultures. This book provides an excellent vehicle to maintain and reinforce this naturally occurring momentum of staff engagement.

Through using a rigorous research methodology, the authors present strong evidence of a link between various highly desirable NHS outcomes and running NHS organizations in certain ways. For instance, NHS organizations that promote and value innovation, staff development and empowerment are likely to be three star trusts. Whilst to some this might not be surprising, it provides the hard evidence that is needed to demonstrate that the 'soft stuff' (i.e. culture) is contingently linked to tangible performance outcomes.

Following on from this theme, organizational culture is as much a prerequisite of NHS failure as it is fundamental to the success of health care. Since the inception of the NHS, more than 30 NHS public inquiries have been conducted to address failures in the quality of care. It is intriguing (and disturbing) that the same common themes can be identified in each report over a 30 year period, from the 1969 Ely Hospital inquiry report on long-stay care for the elderly and mentally ill to the Bristol Royal Infirmary inquiry report on paediatric cardiac surgery published in 2001 (see Higgins 2001; Walshe and Higgins 2002). These common themes are cultural in nature. That is, they include factors such as inadequate managerial and clinical leadership, poor communication and disempowerment of staff and service users.

Solutions to cultural problems have historically been indirectly focused. That is, new structures, systems and procedures are introduced in the hope that they will indirectly deliver changes in organizational culture (i.e. changes in behaviour and mindsets). Whilst structural reforms are important and necessary, they are not sufficient in themselves to deliver improvements in the quality of health care, with services for staff and patients often only changing a little.

Whilst the NHS talks culture change, there is little practical guidance available on how to deliver culture change on the ground. Culture change is assumed to be a natural by-product of the many service improvement initiatives that are currently underway in many health care organizations. Often, these initiatives do not attempt to explicitly understand or address the cultural difficulties that NHS organizations face. Cultural transformation is more likely to emerge from direct attempts to understand and influence the unique unwritten rules and behaviours that heavily influence the work of NHS organizations, as well as indirect attempts.

This book highlights some important 'cultural catalysts', that is, it provides important guidance for organizations on where to focus their energy in order to maximize behavioural and attitudinal change. Mannion, Davies and Marshall found that in high performing NHS organizations:

- leadership is paramount;

- middle managers are strong and empowered;
- high quality information systems underpin robust accountability systems;
- an active human resources function provides the foundations of a performance-conducive culture; and
- high quality inter-relationships with the local health economy are regarded as important.

The experience of the NHS Clinical Governance Support Team reinforces the importance of these characteristics. The team has worked with several organizations that appear to have successfully turned around their dominant culture and attempted to 'bottle the lightening', that is, try to capture the essence of what has made a difference to patients and staff. Specifically, these organizations:

- Understand that the core business of leadership is culture change. Therefore, culture and leadership are regarded as two sides of the same coin.
- In addition to the senior leaders of an organization, those leaders who are dispersed throughout the trust are seen to provide important leverage in managing cultural shifts.
- Fundamentally, the leaders in these organizations understand the paramount importance of consistency between leadership rhetoric and action in bringing about successful culture change.
- They recognize that before leaders can lead others they have to lead themselves. That is, they need to be aware of how their own personality preferences, interpersonal needs, assumptions and behaviours impact upon others within the organization.
- They understand that more often than not organizational inertia is the product of self-limiting beliefs and assumptions as opposed to constraints that are externally imposed to continually monitor their culture.
- They constantly take the cultural 'pulse' of the organization and, where appropriate, work towards challenging the unwritten rules that are at the heart of the way things are done within their organization.
- They value the importance of team work. That is, they recognize the fundamental importance of working well as a management or clinical team if they are to deliver culture change and understand the impact that group dynamics can have on either enabling or inhibiting team effectiveness:
- They use culture change as a 'hook' or a 'driver' to resolve 'live' issues that are pertinent to the future viability of the trust.

- They involve and take into account the needs, fears and motivations of staff at all levels in direction setting and implementation.
- They align their culture change strategies with other improvement
  initiatives.

There is a view that understanding organizational culture does not
matter and intervening in the 'soft and fluffy stuff' is pointless. This
book clearly and empirically refutes this perspective and makes an
invaluable and timely contribution towards understanding and influencing the informal psychological and social aspects of life in the
NHS.

Professor Aidan Halligan
Deputy Chief Medical Officer
Director of Clinical Governance for the NHS

Dr Jay Bevington
Associate Director
NHS Clinical Governance Support Team

FOREWORD BY
NIGEL EDWARDS

Across the world, health care often fails to meet the legitimate expectations of many of its stakeholders. A (relatively limited) battery of (largely structural) solutions are tried, often in rotation, to improve performance – including restructuring, incentives, planning, markets, decentralization, centralization, competing purchasers, managed care and many others. The contradictory nature of many of these prescriptions attests to the popularity of developing interventions without sufficient time being spent on diagnosis. What is more, none of these strategies seems to deliver what is hoped for. To put it another way, health policy and health care management are rich in prescriptions but impoverished in terms of underpinning theory to guide more subtle and effective approaches.

The frustration of managers, policy makers and enthusiasts for quality improvement, is that – despite compelling evidence about the need for change, some pockets of excellence and a considerable body of knowledge about what sort of changes would produce better results for all concerned – health care organizations are often slow to adopt new practices. Health care systems resolutely refuse to do what they are told.

As a result some policy thinkers have changed tack, leading to a great deal of interest in ideas from two related fields: complexity theory and organizational culture. Like many of the more interesting innovations in health care, these ideas have their genesis in disciplines outside of management: in this case biology and social anthropology. Both are promising areas for examination, and both provide a useful antidote for the surprisingly large number of commentators who still hold to the idea that there are simple solutions to complex health care problems.

Both concepts (complexity and culture) were important underpinnings of the Institute of Medicine's (2000) influential *Crossing the
Quality Chasm* report. Perhaps as a result, culture change is now
frequently referred to in policy documents and speeches. Changing
the culture (it is thought) will provide the engine for change, modify
the behaviour of providers and create new and safer environments
for patients and staff. Yet this is a somewhat circular argument as it
does not explain how this culture change will come about, or why
such change will produce the anticipated effects.

Health care management practitioners have learnt their trade
through experience and have no particular underlying theory on
which to hang ideas such as culture change. There is therefore a great
hunger for better ways of conceptualizing the management task, but
unfortunately complex ideas are too often embraced rather too
enthusiastically. As a result many of the caveats, qualifications and
subtleties are often lost in turning ideas into practice.

The analysis in this book shows that the notion of culture needs to
be handled with care. Whilst it has great value as a way of understanding organizational dynamics, there is no n-step procedure by
which culture can be changed to suit the requirements of policy
makers. Indeed, cultures may prove highly resistant to attempts at
change, and even when change does occur there is no particular
guarantee that the result will be higher performance or indeed that
the change will play out anything like that which was intended.
Simplistic attempts to change the culture may have a whole range of
unanticipated and potentially hazardous consequences. A second
important lesson is that talking about a single culture is generally a
mistake. We need to develop a much better understanding of subgroups and subcultures, and the interactions between these. Perhaps
even more significant is the challenge to simple notions of causal
links between culture and organizational performance.

The study identifies a number of important cultural determinants
that seem to contribute to aspects of high performance. Readers
might want to ask themselves whether the current ways of doing
business, existing policy frameworks and the expectations placed on
leaders are sufficiently supportive of the types of behaviour that are
being sought. There are encouraging signs of improvement, but a
number of worrying issues remain:

• First, whilst the importance of leadership is recognized there is
  still a concern that there is an over-emphasis on an inappropriate
  heroic model. The high turnover of chief executives in the NHS

may suggest that the process of defining what sort of management and leadership style is needed by an organization could be improved.

- Second, the status, training and protection given to middle management remain major concerns. Whilst it is this group of managers who seem to be the subject of greatest complaint from doctors, on the positive side NHS staff do seem to appreciate their line managers more than staff in other sectors.
- Third, the finding from this study that inter-relationships with the health economy are important is very significant. Unfortunately many of the incentives, accountabilities and performance management arrangements tend to encourage strategies that maximize individual organizations' goals rather than those of the systems in which they participate.
- Finally, the alignment of objectives at different levels of the organization is clearly seen to be important, but in many health care systems there is a disjunction between the clinical and managerial world and some hostility and lack of comprehension. The way targets are set and performance is managed has tended to make relationships in this area more difficult. Culture is often robust, but when undergoing change new cultural attributes can be fragile: regulation and performance management, for example, can undermine efforts to create positive change.

This book explores the messy, complex and important nature of cultures in health care, together with their relationships with performance. Whilst offering insight and hope, it also provides a timely reminder of the dangers inherent in the over-eager application of simplistic policy remedies.

Nigel Edwards
Policy Director
NHS Confederation

ACKNOWLEDGEMENTS

Contributions to this book were made by: Tim Scott (literature reviewing), Rowena Jacobs (statistical analysis), Alison Powell (assistance with national survey and acute case studies), Liz Nelson (assistance with primary care case studies), Claire-Louise Hodges (assistance with data handling).

Our thanks and acknowledgements for advice and support go to Maria Goddard, Peter C. Smith, Stephen Shortell, Ruth Miller, Liz Brodie and Helen Parkinson. We would particularly like to thank all those from the NHS and associated organizations who gave so freely of their time and insights during every phase of this project. And we would also like to express our gratitude to the Department of Health for the funding of this project – project grant 104R01765 – and core funding for the Centre for Health Economics, University of York, and the National Primary Care Research and Development Centre (NPCRDC), University of Manchester.

INTRODUCTION: POLICY BACKGROUND AND OVERVIEW

POLICY CONTEXT AND POLICY CHANGE

Throughout the 1990s a series of high profile failures in professional practice, most notably the tragic events at Bristol Royal Infirmary (Kennedy 2001), propelled the quality and safety of NHS care up the political agenda. Analysis of these manifest service failings sharpened policy focus on 'modernizing' the deep-seated assumptions, values and working practices that have been affirmed over decades and woven into the fabric of health care delivery. These assumptions, values and patterns of behaviour within an organization are often termed its 'organizational culture' – and it was towards changing this culture that much subsequent health policy effort has been directed.

Such interest is not confined to the United Kingdom: there is increasing international interest in managing organizational culture as a lever for health care improvement. To change the organizational culture alongside structural reforms has become a familiar prescription for health system reform. In the United States, in the wake of high profile reports on medical errors (Institute of Medicine 1999), policy thinking is embracing the notion of culture change as a key element of system redesign (Institute of Medicine 2000). Many other OECD countries are also focusing on cultural renewal as a potential lever for health care quality and performance improvement (Smith 2002). However, it is in the UK National Health Service (NHS) that interest in organizational culture, and initiatives to transform the same, have been most intense.

This interest in culture is not entirely new. Many previous policy reforms in the NHS have also invoked the notion of culture change through attempts to instil new values and modes of working in the organization. Almost 20 years ago the reforms inspired by the Griffiths Report led to the development of general management in hospitals and the greater involvement of clinicians in budgeting and financial matters through a series of resource management initiatives (DHSS 1984). Much of the logic underpinning these changes was extended by the internal market reforms a decade later (Le Grand *et al.* 1998). Central to these reforms were attempts to strengthen managerial control and accountability in the NHS and to nurture a competitive 'business culture' throughout the organization (Davies and Mannion 1999). However, resistance and resilience to these changes was more evident than a wholesale transformation of professional values and behaviour (Broadbent *et al.* 1992; Jones and Dewing 1997).

When elected in 1997 the new Labour government made quality and performance improvement the central reform issues in the NHS (Goddard and Mannion 1998). The new strategy for quality was set out in the 1998 White Paper, *The New NHS: Modern, Dependable* (Department of Health 1997) and supporting policy documents (Department of Health 1998; NHS Executive 1998). These reforms comprised a detailed set of interlocking strategies and supporting activities targeted at three levels:

- defining appropriate quality standards;
- delivering health care congruent with these standards;
- monitoring to ensure that uniformly high quality of care is achieved.

In articulating a coherent strategy needed to reinvigorate health care delivery, official documents stressed the inter-linking of three different strands: clinical governance, life-long learning and professional self-regulation. Underpinning and binding each of these was the notion of cultural transformation as a primary driver for quality improvement:

> . . . achieving meaningful and sustainable quality improvements in the NHS requires a fundamental shift in *culture*, to focus effort where effort is needed and to enable and empower those who work in the NHS to improve quality locally . . . Clinical governance needs to be underpinned by a *culture* that values lifelong learning and recognises the key part it plays in improving quality.
>
> (Department of Health 1998: paragraphs 5.6 and 3.28)

In 2001, the highly influential report published by the Public Inquiry into Children's Heart Surgery at the Bristol Royal Infirmary (Kennedy 2001) concluded that the culture of health care in the NHS 'which so critically affects all other aspects of the service which patients receive, must develop and change'. It described the prevailing culture at the Bristol Royal Infirmary at the time of the tragic events as a 'club culture', which focused excessive power and influence around a core group of senior managers.[1] The report concluded 'the inadequacies in management were an underlying factor which adversely affected the quality and adequacy of care which children received' (Kennedy 2001: 203). Kennedy recognized that while some problems were specific to Bristol, in many ways the Bristol experience exemplified what were and are national issues in the NHS. He then proceeded to pinpoint, with clinical accuracy, the cultural characteristics of the NHS that had colluded in fostering a climate where dysfunctional behaviour and malpractice were not effectively challenged. In making recommendations Kennedy highlighted a number of cultural shifts seen as necessary to transform the NHS into a high quality, safety focused institution, one that was sensitive and responsive to the needs of patients.

The government largely accepted the findings and recommendations of the Bristol Inquiry, and in its published response the Department of Health announced a range of new measures and supporting tactics aimed at tackling the systemic problems identified in the Bristol report (Department of Health 2001a). These included the setting up of a National Patient Safety Agency; a new independent body – the Council for the Regulation of Health Care Professionals, charged with strengthening and co-ordinating the piecemeal system of professional self-regulation; and further release to the public of clinical outcome data (outcomes data were already made publicly available under the performance assessment framework, but this was now extended to individual level data, starting with risk-adjusted mortality rates for all cardiac surgeons in England).

Alongside the reforms outlined above (designed to improve clinical quality, safety and performance) the government also set in train a series of radical changes designed to devolve greater authority and decision-making power to patients and frontline staff. The package of reforms as set out in *The NHS Plan* (Department of Health 2000a) and *Shifting the Balance of Power* documentation (Department of Health 2001b) made clear that cultural change needed to be wrought alongside structural and procedural reform if the anticipated benefits were to be realized. The key challenges as set out in accompanying documentation included (Department of Health 2001c: 2):

- empowering front line staff to use their skills and knowledge to develop innovative services with more say in how services are delivered and resources allocated;
- empowering patients to become informed and active partners in their care involving them in the design, delivery and development of local services;
- changing the NHS culture and structure by devolving power and decision making to frontline staff and primary care trusts (PCTs), and by building clinical networks across organizations.

More recently, health policy in England has seen a revisiting of market incentives and an embracing of 'new localism', including devolution of control through 'earned autonomy'. The principle of earned autonomy is that the highest performing organizations are subject to less central control, have lighter touch scrutiny procedures, and can gain automatic access to funds for which a bidding process would normally apply. One consequence of such an approach has been the introduction of a new type of organization – NHS foundation trusts – that can escape from the vertical hierarchies of control emanating from the Department of Health (Department of Health 2002a, b). A primary tool for deciding on eligibility for various levels of earned autonomy are the NHS performance ratings, which award various 'star ratings' (zero to three) to existing NHS trusts (Department of Health 2002b, 2003; Mannion et al. 2003, 2004). Indeed, policy stipulations dating from 2003 (Department of Health 2003) suggest that all NHS hospitals should be demonstrating the high levels of performance needed to make them eligible for foundation status. It is clear from supporting policy documents that the government expects behavioural changes – especially around innovation, service redesign and customer care – to result from such a freeing up from central control.

The current policy agenda thus highlights cultural change (broadly defined) as one means (alongside structural and procedural reform) of bringing about improvements in health service performance. Yet in any consideration of the role of organizational culture in facilitating high quality and performance in the NHS it is necessary not only to explain what is meant by 'organizational culture' but also to consider what *evidence* there is that organizational culture is linked to performance in meaningful ways within health care delivery organizations.

UNDERLYING LOGIC OF CULTURAL PRESCRIPTIONS

Seeking performance improvement through cultural renewal (intrinsic to many of the recent changes in the NHS) assumes the following stepwise logic:

1 The NHS and its constituent organizations possess a discernible culture or (more likely) cultures.
2 The nature of such cultures has some bearing on performance and quality.
3 Such cultures are malleable and not impervious to purposeful change.
4 It is possible to identify specific cultural attributes that are facilitative of high performance (or at least pinpoint those characteristics which are damaging).
5 Policy makers and managers can design a mix of strategies that can influence the formation of beneficial cultures.
6 The benefits that accrue from managed culture change will outweigh any dysfunctional consequences.

For current policy directions to be well-founded therefore, each of these assumptions would benefit from empirical investigation – to reassure of its substance, and to inform operationalization within the NHS. It is to this end that the work reported here was directed.

AIMS AND OBJECTIVES OF THE STUDY

The overall aim of the project was to investigate, through literature work and empirical study, the extent to which the step-wise logic set out above is supported. In particular, we wished to identify and explicate any possible linkages between the culture(s) of NHS organizations and aspects of their performance, both measured and unmeasured. Key objectives included:

• exploring any empirical relationship(s) between the culture(s) of NHS trusts and their measured (and unmeasured) performance;
• identifying aspects of culture that are seen as targets for managed change, and describing the strategies being employed by organizations to achieve this;
• identifying the levers and facilitators of culture change in health care organizations, and highlighting the key barriers and inhibitors to culture change;

- identifying any contextual factors (e.g. national health policies) that facilitate (or inhibit) the development of virtuous cultures in NHS trusts;
- documenting any unintended and dysfunctional consequences of culture change programmes.

RESEARCH DESIGN AND PROJECT OVERVIEW

While performance and its attainment are central to economics, the study of the policies, institutions and human interactions that underpin it are also the focus of many other disciplines. Thus this project was avowedly *inter-disciplinary* from its inception. In developing the project, the research team drew on expertise, literature, theory and methodologies from economics, management and organization studies, sociology, social psychology, social anthropology, policy studies and health services research.

The aim of the study was to explore the nature of any linkages between organizational culture(s) and performance(s) in the NHS. Given the tremendous methodological difficulties in trying to capture such relationships (not least the problems involved in specifying either culture or performance, and the difficulties of inferring the direction of causality in any uncovered relationships) the project was designed from the outset as a multi-method. In essence, the project consisted of four distinct but inter-related aspects:

1 Stakeholder consultations together with a literature review of both the conceptual underpinnings of organizational culture and extant empirical work examining any culture/performance link in health care.
2 Quantitative assessment of any cross-sectional relationships between senior management team culture and organizational performance in all English acute hospital organizations (NHS acute trusts).
3 Investigation, through intensive multi-method case studies, of the development, maintenance and impact of organizational culture in six NHS acute sector health care organizations.
4 Investigation, through intensive multi-method case studies, of the development, maintenance and impact of organizational culture in six NHS primary care health care organizations.

A detailed explanation of the methods is given in Appendix 1; the remainder of the text reports the conceptual and empirical findings from each part of the study. Chapter 1 explores in some depth the multi-disciplinary roots of notions of organization culture, the relevance of these to understanding health care delivery, and the associated issues of cultural change and leadership. Chapter 2 examines previous published empirical work on any culture/performance linkages to assess the extent of the extant evidence base and the lessons that can be drawn from this for future study. The next four chapters present the main findings from fresh empirical study in the NHS: first, from in-depth case study work in selected English NHS acute trusts (Chapters 3 and 4), then from a national quantitative assessment of culture/performance linkages in all English NHS acute trusts (Chapter 5), finally from an examination of culture/performance dynamics in six selected primary care trusts (Chapter 6). The book concludes (Chapter 7) with both an examination of the policy implications of these findings and a look forward at the emerging research agenda around these issues.

NOTE

1 In referring to a 'club culture' the Kennedy Report was invoking a cultural typology reported by Charles Handy (Handy 1988). Here the central individuals of an organization are seen as behaving like a club of like-minded individuals. At the centre are one (or a few) very influential 'rulers' (Handy likens these to Zeus, principal god of the Greek pantheon, and prone to personal and capricious interventions). In club cultures, lines of influence are much more important than lines of accountability.

1

MAKING SENSE OF ORGANIZATIONAL CULTURE IN HEALTH CARE
(with Tim Scott)

INTRODUCTION

Modern health care policy frequently invokes notions of 'cultural change' as a key means of achieving performance improvement and good health care quality. Questions then arise as to whether this is largely empty rhetoric – a convenient shorthand for radical change – or whether this framing of health care organizations in 'cultural' terms offers a useful means of understanding and managing, with the potential for beneficial improvements in both the processes and the outcomes of care.

This chapter begins the process of unpacking what is meant by 'organizational culture'. It introduces some of the sources of ideas, conceptual underpinnings and key concerns with using notions of organizational culture, before considering the relationship between organizational culture, organizational change and leadership. First however, we begin our inter-disciplinary tour with a review of culture in economic thought. We use economics as our point of departure to emphasize and clarify that an understanding of culture is indeed central to an understanding of organizational performance.

CULTURE IN ECONOMIC THOUGHT

An extension of economists' thinking – to acknowledge the significance of culture in all its aspects in human affairs, and to consider the implications and ramifications of the linkages between economic and cultural systems – would seem to be essential if the science of economics is to deal adequately with the contemporary condition.

(Throsby 2001: 165–6)

Economists working within the mainstream (neoclassical) tradition have tended to downplay the importance of cultural factors in framing economic decisions, shaping preferences, driving motivations and regulating behaviour. Nevertheless, culture lurks near the surface of neoclassical thought: as Smelser (1992: 23) notes, 'the idea of rational choice is indeed an idea of culture, however thin that idea might be'.

Neoclassical economists prefer to conceive of economic behaviour as the outcome of fixed and universal human traits that transcend particular social settings. According to Becker 'all human behaviour can be viewed as involving participants who maximize their utility from a stable set of preferences' (Becker 1976: 14). Thus, the neoclassical economist has little to say about the formation of wants and preferences (these are viewed as the province of sociologists and psychologists) and the aim of the economist is to trace the consequences of any given set of *exogenously* determined preferences. If culture matters, however, preference patterns for the same individual may differ across cultural settings and therefore their preferences will be *endogenously* determined.

The lack of realism contained in the neoclassical approach has traditionally been defended on the grounds that it is the predictive power of the model that counts, not the realism of its behavioural assumptions (Machlup 1981). Here it is useful to introduce Gudeman's (1986) distinction between what he refers to as the 'universalist' approach to economic explanation on the one hand and the 'localist' approach on the other. Universalism implies that economic explanations or models apply to the description of economic activity in all places at all times (also see Katzner 2002). From the localist perspectives, however, an individual's behaviour is explained only on the basis of their own understandings of the reality that surrounds them (e.g. nationally or organizationally) and thus those understandings are defined in terms of the cultural patterns within which those agents are situated.

The view that economic models predicated on universalist assumptions can yield any insights into complex economic systems fuelled by endogenously changing preferences is increasingly under attack – not least by evolutionary and institutional economists (Lindbeck 1995; Bowles 1998; Fuchs 2000). There have also been calls for the development of approaches that better reflect the contingent and learned nature of economic action, and which allow for an appreciation of the ways in which economic behaviour is shaped by the dynamic inter-play of the constraining and liberating effects of culture bearing milieus (Mannion and Small 1999). Indeed, according to Mayhew (1994), it was the application of the concept of culture to economic processes that created institutional economics as a separate intellectual tradition.

INSTITUTIONS, PREFERENCE FORMATION AND ECONOMIC CO-ORDINATION

In institutional economics the main foci of study are the 'habits of use' and 'institutions' that taken together form the patterns of a culture. Here, institutions are taken as the 'rules of the game in a society' or in more prosaic terms the 'humanly devised constraints that shape human interaction and structure incentives in human exchange' (North 1990). In considering institutions, it is standard to distinguish between those that are external and those that are internal (see Box 1.1) – with internal institutions transmitted,

---

Box 1.1   Institutions and economic theory

Institutions can be defined as human-devised *rules* that constrain possibly arbitrary and opportunistic behaviour in human interaction. Institutions are shared in a community and are enforced by some sort of sanction. Institutions can economize on the costs of finding and processing relevant knowledge and on transacting business. When institutions are poorly defined or authorities complicate the rule system, institutions can suffer from dysfunctional complexity.

Internal institutions evolve from human experience and incorporate solutions that have tended to serve people best in the past. Examples are customs, ethical norms, manners and trade conventions. Violations of internal institutions tend to be sanctioned informally.

External institutions are imposed and enforced from above, having been designed and established by agents who are authorized by a political process. External institutions are coupled with explicit sanctions, which are imposed in formal ways and may be enforced by the legitimated use of force.

Box 1.2 Different types of internal institutions

We can distinguish four broad, though overlapping, categories of internal institutions which differ in the way in which adherence is monitored and breaches are sanctioned:

- *Conventions* are rules that are so obviously convenient that people self-enforce, by and large, out of self-interest.
- *Internalized rules* arise where people have learnt the rules by habit, education or experience, so that the rules are normally obeyed spontaneously and without reflection.
- *Customs and good manners* represent a third type of internal institution. Violations do not automatically attract organized sanctions, but others in the community tend to supervise rule compliance informally, and violators may find themselves excluded.
- *Formalized internal rules* represent the final type. Here, rules have emerged with experience, but they are formally monitored and enforced. Communities create much law internally but then enforce it among themselves in organized ways through third parties. These may be adjudicators (people who clarify the rules and spell out possible sanctions) and arbitrators (third parties who make binding decisions on interpretation and sanctions).

Source: Derived and adapted from Kasper and Streit (1998)

---

embedded and enforced via a web of overlapping and interconnected cultural processes (see Box 1.2).

One function of 'institutions' is to make the complex processes of human interaction more understandable and predictable so that co-ordination between different individuals occurs more readily. In this way institutions affect the performance of the economy by their effect on the costs of production and exchange. Together with the technology deployed they determine the transaction and transformation costs that make up total economic costs (Kasper and Streit 1998). Therefore, the institutional basis of a society constitutes an important part of that society's social capital and holds important implications for how effectively physical and human resources are put to work (Coleman 1990).

Recent work has explored the influence economic institutions and their attendant cultures have on the formation of individual preferences. For example Bowles (1998) in his article, Endogenous preferences: the cultural consequences of markets and other economic institutions, identifies five mediating cultural effects of economic institutions and explores their influence on the evolution of values, tastes and preferences. These are discussed in outline below.

1 *Framing and situational construal*: economic institutions are 'situations' in a social-psychological sense and thus possess framing and situation construal effects. Therefore a choice problem presented in a market environment may induce behaviours different from the identical problem framed in a non-market way.

2 *Intrinsic and extrinsic motivations*: the reward systems of different institutions may affect motivation independently of framing effects. For example an external institution may *crowd out* intrinsic motivation when it is perceived to be controlling but *crowds in* intrinsic motivation when it is perceived to be supporting self-determination and self-esteem. Controlled experimental work in psychology (Deci and Ryan 1987) has shown that the *crowding out* effect (in other words the institution is perceived as controlling) is stronger where:
   • the rewards are expected (unexpected rewards have a weaker or even no negative effect on intrinsic motivation);
   • the rewards are most salient;
   • the rewards are contingent on task completion or on performance;
   • deadlines and threats are used alongside intensive surveillance.

3 *Effects on the evolution of norms*: economic institutions influence the structure of social interactions and thus affect the evolution of norms by altering the expected benefits to relationships. For example the impersonal and ephemeral nature of market transactions may place less demands on people's 'elevated motivations' and therefore affect the costs and benefits of acquiring cultural traits affecting socially desirable behaviours (e.g. altruism, trustworthiness or compassion).

4 *Task performance effects*: economic institutions structure the tasks people face and therefore influence not only their capacities but their values and psychological functioning as well.

5 *Effects of the process of cultural transmission*: markets and other institutions affect the cultural learning process itself and may alter the ways values and beliefs are acquired and generated from one generation to another. The analysis applies equally to the transmission of core cultural traits to new generations of employees within an organization over a period of time.

Bowles (1998) also points out that there is growing evidence to suggest that preferences learned or internalized under one set of circumstances may become generalized to another. Thus for example a specific economic institution may induce self-regarding and opportunistic behaviour that then becomes part of the behavioural repertoire of that individual. This suggests that certain economic institutions may generate a form of behavioural stickiness, which is hard to dislodge even when institutional structures are changed dramatically.

AN ECONOMIC PERSPECTIVE ON 'CORPORATE' CULTURE

Taking an institutional economic perspective admits the possibility that an organization's 'corporate identity' and core values help mould its members' preference patterns – and hence influences their economic behaviour. It is therefore possible to speculate that an organization's culture may affect economic performance in at least four directions (Kreps 1990; Hodgson 1996; Carrillo and Gromb 1999; Hermalin 2000; Throsby 2001; Smith *et al.* 2003):

1 Culture may drive economic *efficiency*, via the promotion of shared values and internalized norms within the organization, which in turn condition the ways in which the group's members engage and co-operate in the processes of production and exchange. Specific cultural values may be more or less conducive to (for example): effective decision making; reporting and learning from mistakes; team-based working; interdepartmental synergies; creativity; and more adaptive behaviour in making internal changes in response to changes in the external environment.

2 Culture may affect *equity*, for example by inculcating shared moral principles of concern for others, and establishing organizational mechanisms that foster departures from purely efficiency-seeking behaviour.

3 Culture may influence the overall *economic and social objectives* that an organization pursues. Thus, the corporate culture may be one of concern for employees and their working conditions and these values may mitigate the importance of surplus seeking, market share or other economic goals in the organization's objective function. Alternatively, some senior management

cultures may value achieving externally set performance targets over the quality of the working lives of staff, or value their attainment more highly than areas of organizational performance that are not monitored by external agencies.

4 Finally, where the interaction between agents is extremely complex – and difficult for either party to monitor the actions of their counterparts – corporate culture may encourage *co-operation* and relationship building among agents (intra- and inter-organizational partnership working). The process works through the creation and maintenance of *reputation*, where both parties signal their commitment to co-operation by articulating and adhering to identifiable sets of values.

INSTITUTIONS AND GOVERNANCE

Ouchi (1979, 1980) addressed a similar issue in developing a simple economic model to relate modes of governance to efficient production. He posits that the choice over the most efficient economic governance or institutional structure for the production of a given good or service is linked to the ease by which outputs can be measured and the degree of clarity of understanding of the transformation process by which inputs are transformed into outputs. These issues give rise to three possible institutional options (see Table 1.1).

Where outputs are easily measurable, but knowledge of the transformation process is imperfect, it may be more efficient to use a market system where all relevant information is captured in the clearing price. Where outputs are not easily measured but the transformation process is well understood, knowledge of the behaviour of those involved in the transformation process is the key informational requirement. In this case the more efficient mode of control may the use of hierarchical institutions that rely on prescribed rules and

Table 1.1 Efficient economic governance frameworks and antecedent conditions

Ability to measure outputs	*Knowledge of the transformation process*	
	Perfect	*Imperfect*
High	Markets/hierarchies	Markets
Low	Hierarchies	Culture

Source: adapted from Ouchi (1980)

targets, enforced by surveillance of subordinates by superiors in the hierarchy (e.g. by use of performance indicators, and ensuring adherence to guidelines). In the case where it is possible to measure outputs easily and where the transformation process is understood either markets or hierarchies are suitable modes of governance. Where the opposite scenario exists and it is not easy to measure outputs and the transformation process is not well understood (as is the case with many health and clinical services), Ouchi identifies the importance of social or cultural controls and the associated 'clan' governance.

In Ouchi's notion of 'clan culture' members share a common (often professional) culture. Individuals are socialized into particular traditions regarding appropriate behaviour and develop a high commitment to a code of conduct. Rewards are attached to displaying the correct attitudes and values and these may be expressed in the form of rituals or ceremonies that in turn serve to reinforce the same attitudes and values. Performance information is transmitted *via* soft and informal channels and is closely associated with the standards and norms of professional behaviour. Clearly the medical profession exhibit many of the classic traits of an internal institution. Clinicians, through their professional training and specialized knowledge, are best placed to understand the transformation process and assessment of performance has traditionally been *via* systems of professional regulation, peer review and audit.

In sum organizational or corporate culture may be viewed usefully as both a complement and a substitute for many of the other governance structures economists have studied, and by extension the cultures of health care organizations may be expected to be intimately related to their economic performance. However, while culture can be seen to underpin many economic phenomena (including performance), its *unpacking* – understanding its source, development, maintenance and ramifications – has by and large been addressed more fully by sociologists and social anthropologists. It is this literature that we explore next.

UNDERSTANDING ORGANIZATIONAL CULTURE

In his seminal monograph, *Leadership in Administration* (1957), Philip Selznick distinguishes between two ideal types in any collective enterprise: on the one hand, there is a rational instrumental *organization*, and on the other there exists a value-infused *mini-society*.[1] In the mechanistic 'organization', tasks are allocated, authority delegated, communications channelled and the whole enterprise can be seen in terms of co-ordinating and rationing out of work. The mini-society, in contrast but intertwined with the mechanistic organization, is an organic social entity, infused with values and emerging from natural social processes. Thus, to understand social and commercial enterprises, we need to address both of these aspects. It is the latter – *the value-infused mini-society* – which is the domain of organizational culture studies.

Organizational culture is an anthropological metaphor, one of many metaphors used to inform research, consultancy and management in organizations (Morgan 1986). Early in the twentieth century, social anthropologists described processes of socialization in societies through family, community, educational, religious and other institutions (Williams 1983). That these ideas have some relevance for organizational study can be traced back at least as far as the Hawthorne studies and related work (Roethlisberger and Dixon 1939). Those studies observed how the informal, *social* dimension of enterprise mediated between organizational structures and performance, and how these aspects could be manipulated to affect employee effort and commitment. In the post-war period a number of researchers, including behavioural economists (Cyert and March 1963), industrial sociologists (Selznick 1957), organizational psychologists (Schein 1985a, b) and others (Allaire and Firsirotu 1984), have emphasized the importance of culture in shaping organizational behaviour and hence economic performance.

DEFINITIONS OF ORGANIZATIONAL CULTURE

The key methodological principle in studies of organizational culture is to investigate organizations as mini-societies (Allaire and Firsirotu 1984; Ashkanasy and Jackson 2001). They aim to illuminate participants' interpretations, evaluations and expressions of their roles within the social, political and technical life-world of an organization. However, there is little consensus among scholars over the precise meaning of *organizational culture*; a plethora of definitions of organizational culture can be found in the literature (Ott 1989; Alvesson 1995; Brown 1995), and some of the underlying foci of these are outlined in Table 1.2. Most of these definitions implicitly recognize the socially constructed nature of the phenomenon, locate its generation in pervasive, normative beliefs and values, and see its

Table 1.2 Conceptions of organizational culture

Focus	Description
Exchange regulation	A form of control used to shape shared views with a view to reducing transaction costs.
Compass	A shared value system that provides guidance and direction.
Social glue	The shared values, beliefs, understandings and norms that bind an organization's members into collective endeavour.
Sacred cow	Ideals and values internalized and held sacred by an organization's members.
Management control	The manipulation of beliefs and values as a means of meeting strategic objectives.
Affect regulation	The control and management of the affective and expressive elements of organization.
Non-order	The inherent ambiguity, uncertainty, contradiction and confusion of organizational life.
Blinders	The deep aspects that provide an unconscious guide to behaviour.
World closure	A shared view on life.
Dramaturgical domination	The manipulation of symbols and their dramatic attributes in a political context.

Source: Abstracted from Alvesson (1995)

expression in terms of patterns of behaviour. For these reasons, the definition we find most helpful, and that which underpins the thinking in this study, is that developed by Schein, who defined organizational culture as:

> the pattern of shared basic assumptions – invented, discovered or developed by a given group as it learns to cope with its problems of external adaptation and internal integration – that has worked well enough to be considered valid and, therefore, to be taught to new members as the correct way to perceive, think, and feel in relation to those problems.
>
> (Schein 1985b)

Arguably, then, what essentially distinguishes one culture from another is their varying and vast pools of tacit knowledge – which natives understand but are not necessarily conscious of knowing. Culture, therefore, is not merely the observable in social life, it is also the shared cognitive and symbolic context within which a society or institution can be understood.

ORGANIZATIONAL CULTURE AND ORGANIZATIONAL CLIMATE

Organizational culture is related to – and sometimes conceptually rather indistinct from – organizational climate (a meteorological metaphor). Although culture and climate have much in common, and are often used with unclear delineation (Schneider 1990; Denison 1996; Payne 2000; Ashkanasy and Jackson 2001; Bower *et al.* 2003), studies of culture attempt to access deeper values and assumptions rather than the surface perceptions that are the focus of climate studies (Denison 1996; Payne 2000; Schein 2000). Organizational culture also emphasizes that which is shared by group members (Davies *et al.* 2000), and is more concerned with a qualitative understanding within a particular social setting, an understanding that emphasizes the historical dynamics from which the culture emerges, rather than with quantitative snapshots that compare the climate of organizations at a given time point (Fey and Beamish 2001). Nonetheless the overlaps between these two metaphors are significant, and some authors have suggested that variations in use of the terms represent more historical fad and fashion than substantive difference (Schneider and Reichers 1983; Fey and Beamish 2001). Indeed, the term 'climate' is sometimes used by those who are interested in the concepts underlying organizational culture, but who have concerns about the ways in which the term has been abused in the past.

LEVELS OF CULTURE

For all the disputes over the precise definitions of organizational culture, most commentators agree that it is layered in nature. Schein's identification of three levels of ascending importance (Schein 1985b) provides one of the most useful and widely acknowledged frameworks for analysis:

Level 1   *Artefacts* – the most visible manifestations of culture, including its rituals, rewards and ceremonies. Artefacts are especially concerned with observable patterns of behaviour within organizations. In health services these may include such diverse issues as dress codes (the doctors' ubiquitous white coat and tie), standard ways of running services (the physician's beds, the surgeon's list, juniors attached to seniors) or methods of performance assessment (the dominance of confidential peer review, the reliance on professional self-regulation).

Level 2   *Beliefs and values* – espoused beliefs and values which may be used to justify particular behaviour patterns and which form the basis for choosing between alternative courses of action. For example in the medical profession conduct has traditionally been based on the Hippocratic principle of placing the needs of individual patients above broader economic and corporate objectives, this in turn has led to clinical freedom being a highly prized cultural 'value'. Other beliefs and values that may (purportedly) influence behaviour are, for example, a belief in evidence or assertions about patient autonomy.

Level 3   *Assumptions* – the real, unspoken, largely unconscious beliefs, values and expectations held and shared by individuals; these may be signalled by artefacts that belie the espoused beliefs and values. For example medical research has traditionally been predicated on the use of rational scientific methods as the basis of generating and accumulating knowledge (controlled trials rather than qualitative and interpretative methods). Thus assumptions about measurability, aggregation and transferability of knowledge are deeply ingrained in medical care. Similarly, a biomedical (as compared to a biopsychosocial) understanding of health and illness may exert significant (perhaps unnoticed) influence.

For all that these varying levels of culture have been identified and conceptualized, relatively little work to date has succeeded in exploring the deeper levels of culture (Scott *et al.* 2001, 2003a, b). Indeed, work on cultural change suggests that while artefacts may be relatively susceptible to apparently important shifts, the deeper assumptions may remain unchanged with the potential to negate, attenuate or redirect the change effort (Jones and Dewing 1997; Harris and Ogbonna 2002).

COMPETING SCHOOLS OF THOUGHT ON ORGANIZATIONAL CULTURE

Conventionally the culture literature is divided into two broad streams (Smircich 1983). One stream approaches culture as an *attribute*, something an organization *has*, alongside other attributes such as structure and strategy. Another stream of literature regards culture more globally as defining the whole character and experience of organizational life – what the organization *is*. Here organizations are construed as cultures existing in and reproduced through the social interactions of their participants. This may be termed the *culture as metaphor* approach. Key differences between these two approaches are outlined in Table 1.3.

The distinction between viewing culture as either an attribute (a defining quality), or a metaphor, holds important policy implications. The view of culture as an attribute has been instrumentally interpreted as meaning that culture is an independent variable

Table 1.3   Comparing 'culture as an attribute' and 'culture as a metaphor'

	Culture as an attribute	Culture as a metaphor
Disciplinary base	Social psychology	Anthropology
Epistemological assumptions	Positivist	Phenomenological
Methodology	Nomothetic	Ideographic
Theory of cultural cohesion	Unitary culture	Co-existing subcultures
Theory of organizational order	Consensus	Conflict
Creation and transmission of culture	Formed and directed by actions of senior staff to change artefacts and espoused ideology	Reproduced by all culture members through their ongoing social interactions
Culture change agents	Senior management manipulate culture to meet corporate objectives	Managers, as well as other organization members, seek to influence cultural direction of the organization

capable of manipulation to satisfy organizational objectives. From that perspective culture change is viewed as a means to commercial or other technical ends and comprises a range of activities directed at 'overhauling' or 're-engineering' an organization's value system. Much popular management literature adopts that approach (e.g. Peters and Waterman 1982). If, by contrast, organizations are approached as cultural systems (culture as metaphor), then culture becomes the defining context by which the meaning of organizational attributes is revealed. Then, change agents are offered fewer levers to influence the formation of desirable cultures. Indeed the whole emphasis shifts from an economic perspective on *what* organizations can achieve to an anthropological understanding of *how* organizations are socially accomplished and reproduced.

Of course, not all scholars and commentators are enamoured of culture as a means of understanding organizational dynamics. Indeed, post-modern perspectives on organizational culture dispute the very notion of organizations and their cultures as concrete entities (see Box 1.3). Others contend that organizational culture

---

Box 1.3   Post-modern perspectives on organizational culture

Post-modern perspectives are best understood in contrast with modernism. At the core of a modernist approach is a view that organizational phenomena (including cultures, structures and performance) are concrete entities, which can be systematically described and explained. Such modernist accounts have proved immensely influential, not least because they offer managers and policy makers the seductive view that better understanding of this empirical reality will bring improved organizational control and performance. The latest NHS reforms conform to this modernist conception of organizational life, and some of our research approach colludes with this view.

Over recent years however, the modernist position on organization studies been subjected to a sustained critique from a range of loosely coupled approaches that have been termed *post-modern* (Mannion and Small 1999). Although it is difficult to offer a precise definition of the term post-modernism (indeed the post-modern value of diversity precludes this), a number of broad themes can be identified:

- Postmodernism sees the social world as constructed by our shared language, and asserts that we can only 'know' this world through the particular form of discourse our language creates.

- Organizations are not seen as concrete entities, to be revealed through the process of objective and scientific research, but are seen as being socially and discursively constructed. As reflections of a form of discourse (i.e. linguistic artefacts) they are unstable and fragile.
- The task of a post-modern analysis therefore is to deconstruct current processes of sense-making to expose the unstable and superficial nature of social structures and practices, and to reveal the hidden contradictions, tensions and 'unreason' inherent in human experience.

One strand of post-modern analysis is concerned with how what is legitimized as knowledge is governed and constrained by vested interests. Different groups struggle and compete to impose their definitions. Knowledge is what the powerful *say* is knowledge; and those who define what knowledge is, are considered powerful. Therefore, post-modernism aims at understanding how groups engage in struggles to offer an authentic and legitimized view of the world (Foucault 1972). Post-modern perspectives thus encourage a diversity of voices and the celebration of difference (Clegg 1990; Gergen 1992).

A post-modern perspective on organizational culture would not focus on cultures as a means of control. It would instead encourage dialogue on the nature and course of change among stakeholders, particularly those who traditionally have been disfranchised or marginalized from such discussions. The emphasis of such a dialogue would be on challenging existing authorized accounts and balances of power, rather than on the refinement of mechanisms of control.

remains vague as a concept, being defined more by what it is not (structure, process) than what it actually is, and thus remains an *'unexplained catch-all, which appears to offer little of pragmatic value'* (Ormrod 2003). More critical and political perspectives (e.g. Willmott 1993; Alvesson and Willmott 2002) go further to suggest that 'managing culture' involves wholesale appropriation of employees in furtherance of corporate goals and is thus necessarily oppressive in nature.

CULTURE AS EMERGENCE

Different conceptualizations generate rival claims as to the nature and feasibility of planned cultural change, with 'culture as attribute' offering more scope for purposive manipulation than 'culture as metaphor'. However, for the purposes of much of this work we tread a middle path between the two dominant approaches by treating an organization's culture as an emergent property concomitant with its status as a mini-society (Selznick 1957; Douglas 1985). Thus culture is not thought of as something fixed and static, but is seen instead as something which all those in an organization are constantly creating, affirming and expressing:

> Organisational culture is the emergent result of the continuing negotiations about values, meaning and properties between the members of an organisation and with its environment.
>
> (Seel 2000)

By this definition, culture is not assumed *a priori* to be controllable. Instead we consider that its main characteristics can at least be described and assessed in terms of their functional contribution to broader managerial and organizational objectives (including per-formance) (Davies *et al.* 2000). Following from this, brief consider-ation of two examples will help to clarify how use of a 'cultural lens' can shed light onto important aspects of organizational dynamics in health care. We look first at some of the ideas underpinning 'safety cultures' before outlining some of the key attributes of 'learning cultures'.

SAFETY CULTURES IN HEALTH CARE

The Advisory Committee on the Safety of Nuclear Installations defines the safety culture of an organization as 'the product of indi-vidual and group values, attitudes, perceptions, competencies and patterns of behaviour that determine the commitment to, and the style and proficiency of, an organisation's health and safety man-agement' (quoted in Nieva 2002). But concerns with safety are not confined to high-risk areas of industry: there is now clear evidence of significant problems with patient safety in all health care systems that have been examined (Brennan *et al.* 1991; Wilson *et al.* 1995; Vincent *et al.* 2000). As such, patient safety has attracted much attention from policy makers, practitioners and academics in recent years. Two policy documents have been particularly influential in this respect: *To Err is Human* (Kohn *et al.* 2000), published by the Institute of Medicine in the United States and *An Organisation With A Memory* from the UK (Department of Health 2000b). Both of these reports describe how organizational culture can influence the attitudes and behaviour of individual employees and highlight the importance of a systems-based approach to facilitate the development of a culture that promotes safe practice in health organizations.

Policy documents tend to shy away from formal definitions of 'safety cultures', listing instead the key cultural components or dimensions relevant to patient safety. Indeed, there is a high level of agreement amongst commentators about the key features of an organization with an effective safety culture (e.g. Pidgeon 1997; Reason 1997; Weick *et al.* 1999; Nieva 2002; Nieva and Sorra 2003; Singer *et al.* 2003). These are summarized in Box 1.4.

Research into the nature and causes of safety problems in health organizations has identified a number of common cultural problems. First, and most prominent, is the propensity to blame individuals when things go wrong (Department of Health 2001d; Pidgeon 1997; Singer *et al.* 2003). This has been a termed a 'blame culture' and much attention has been focused on the need to develop a 'no blame culture' in health organizations. More recently, however, 'no blame' has been replaced by the phrase 'open and fair' to reflect the fact that sometimes individuals are at fault for errors. Despite the rhetoric about systematic causes for errors, individual blame is still a major barrier to improving safety cultures.

The second problem relates to professional boundaries or 'silos' (Firth-Cozens *et al.* 2002). Neither the traditional 'closing of ranks' of the medical profession, nor the 'scapegoating' of the nursing profession help to produce a culture conducive to safety. Brooks, in a phenomenological study of professional groups in hospitals, described the rituals conducted by professionals that help to preserve or break down traditional boundaries – and so explored the impact of these rituals on safety culture (Brooks and Brown 2002). Others have highlighted the negative impact on safety of the traditional culture of individualism amongst doctors (Caroll *et al.* 2002) and the lack of team-work within hospitals which can contribute to unsafe practices (Singer *et al.* 2003).

The third major problem with the culture in health care with respect to patient safety relates to the traditional methods of learning adopted by most health professionals. In particular, the medical profession has not traditionally practised the reflexivity or self-appraisal that is a fundamental part of learning from mistakes. This is particularly true given the exceptional potential of learning from the so-called 'near misses' that probably account for over 300 times

Box 1.4   Key features of an organization with a 'good' safety culture

Dimension	Components
Effective leadership	Senior management committed to safe practices Concern for impact of hazards on staff and patients Higher value given to safety than productivity Values made explicit
Commitment to continuous learning	Focus on feedback and reflection Encouragement of a questioning attitude amongst staff Celebration of successes
Use of data	Willingness to collect and use data on adverse events and near misses Self-reporting regarded as the norm
Flexibility	Delegation to frontline staff Appropriate use of skills
Just and fair response to adverse events	Creation of a 'no blame' culture Recognition of inter-dependency of systems and individuals in causation and prevention of adverse events Non-punitive response to errors Appropriate attribution when mistakes occur
Effective teamwork	High quality communication within and between teams High value placed on multi-disciplinarity Mutual respect
Openness and honesty	Disclosure of adverse events to patients
Willingness to commit resources	Sufficient staff, time and finances allocated to improving and maintaining safety Effective use of appropriate incentives to improve safety

the number of fatalities and ten times the number of non-fatal events in a health setting (Department of Health 2001d).

Of course, safety cultures are not just a matter of internal organization – they are also a function of the external financial, political and regulatory environment. For example, lack of funding, expectations about long hours worked in training, pressures arising from the public reporting of performance, and the demands of external scrutiny can all have significant impacts. The safety – or otherwise – of the extant culture will be a product of these external factors as well as those aspects of organizational life specific the organization itself.

Thus ideas of 'safety cultures' appear to provide a useful means of developing understanding of the human and organizational dimensions of patient safety. They focus on the values, beliefs and assumptions that underpin patterns of behaviour, especially those concerned with risk-taking and rule violation (Gosbee 2002; Pizzi *et al.* 2003). In doing so, they emphasize the dynamic and complex cognitive processes taking place within and between individuals in organizations, and the inter-connectedness of these with established organizational structures and processes. The need for learning inherent in safety cultures provides a convenient link to consideration of the nature of cultures that support successful learning in organizations.

LEARNING CULTURES IN HEALTH CARE

Learning is something undertaken and developed by individuals, but organizational arrangements can foster or inhibit this learning process: the organizational culture within which individuals work shapes their engagement with the learning process. Organizations that position learning as a core characteristic have been termed 'learning organizations' (Senge 1985; Davies and Nutley 2000). The key features of learning organizations are outlined in Box 1.5. They relate less to the ways in which organizations are structured and more to the ways in which people within the organization think about the nature of, and the relationships between, the outside world, their organization, their colleagues and themselves.

Building learning organizations is in effect an attempt to manage the culture of that organization. Thus it requires attention to some key cultural values if it is to be a successful undertaking. Some of the values most commonly associated with organizational learning are

---

Box 1.5   Key features of a learning organization

Open systems thinking. Individuals within organizations can tend to see activities in a somewhat isolated way, disconnected from the whole. The disease model prevalent in modern health care, which structures services by diseases or procedures, contributes to such isolationism. 'Open systems thinking' encapsulates the notion of teaching people to reintegrate activities, to see how what they do and what others do are inter-connected. This reintegration needs to stretch beyond internal departmental boundaries, and even beyond the boundaries of the organization itself, to encompass other services and patients.

Improving individual capabilities. For an organization to be striving for excellence, the individuals within that organization must constantly be improving their own personal proficiencies. However, separate learning by the different professions in health care may be detrimental because individual virtuosity is insufficient – it is teams that deliver health care.

Team learning. Team learning is vital because it is largely through teams that organizations achieve their objectives. Therefore whole-team development is essential rather than piecemeal uni-professional learning.

Updating mental models. 'Mental models' are the deeply held assumptions and generalizations formed by individuals (internally and often implicitly). These models influence how people make sense of the world. They control, for example, how causes and effects are linked conceptually, and constrain what individuals see as possible within the organization. Changing and updating these mental models is essential to finding new ways of doing things.

A cohering vision. Empowering and enabling individuals within an organization has to be counterbalanced by providing clear strategic direction and articulating a coherent set of values that can guide individual actions. Encouraging a shared understanding of this vision, and commitment to it, is a crucial component of building a learning organization.

Source: Reproduced from Davies and Nutley (2000)

---

outlined in Box 1.6. Some of these values are already central to the health care professions and the NHS (e.g. the celebration of success); others may need more work (e.g. openness and trust).

Thus much of what we currently understand about processes of collective learning (and the retention, sharing and deployment of

Box 1.6 Cultural values underpinning learning organizations

Celebration of success. If excellence is to be pursued with vigour and commitment, its attainment must be valued within the organizational culture.

Absence of complacency. Learning organizations reject the adage 'if it ain't broke don't fix it' – they are searching constantly for new ways of delivering products and services. Thus innovation and change are valued within the organization.

Tolerance of mistakes. Learning from failure is a prerequisite for progressive organizations. This in turn requires a culture that accepts the positive spin-offs from errors, rather than seeks to blame and scapegoat. (This does not, however, imply a tolerance of routinely poor or mediocre performance from which no lessons are learned.)

Belief in human potential. It is people that drive success in organizations – using their creativity, energy and innovation. Therefore the culture within a learning organization values people, and fosters their professional and personal development.

Recognition of tacit knowledge. Learning organizations recognize that those individuals closest to processes have the best and most intimate knowledge about their potential and flaws. Therefore the learning culture values tacit knowledge, and demonstrates a belief in empowerment (the systematic enlargement of discretion, responsibility and competence).

Openness. Because learning organizations try to foster a 'systems' view, sharing knowledge throughout the organization is one key to developing learning capacity. 'Knowledge mobility' emphasizes informal channels and personal contacts over written reporting procedures. Cross-disciplinary and multi-function teams, staff rotations, on-site inspections and experiential learning are essential components of this informal exchange.

Trust. For individuals to give of their best, take risks and develop their competencies, they must trust that such activities will be appreciated and valued by colleagues and managers. In particular, they must be confident that should they err they will be supported not castigated. In turn, managers must be able to trust that subordinates will use wisely the time, space and resources given to them through empowerment programmes – and not indulge in opportunistic behaviour. Without trust, learning is a faltering process.

Outward looking. Learning organizations are engaged with the world outside as a rich source of learning opportunities. They look to their competitors for insights into their own operations and are attuned to the experiences of other stakeholders such as their suppliers. In particular, they are focused on obtaining a deep understanding of clients' needs.

Source: Reproduced from Davies and Nutley (2000)

that learning) draws upon a cultural understanding of health care organizations. We need to understand much more about how the cultural values that underpin learning are developed, maintained, communicated and expressed. In addressing these issues, one important consideration will be how and why cultures vary between groups and subgroups within the organization.

CULTURAL DIVERSITY AND THE ROLE OF SUBCULTURES

The culture found within an organization may be far from uniform or coherent (Martin 1992; Langfield-Smith 1995; Degeling *et al.* 1998). Indeed, looking for commonality may be less rewarding than an examination of differences (see Box 1.7). Although some cultural attributes may be seen across an organization, others may be prominent only in some sections of that organization. Different cultures may emerge, for example, within different occupational or professional groups, and these groups may even seek to differentiate themselves from one another by their cultural artefacts or values. Subcultures are also likely to be associated with different levels of power and influence within the organization, whose dynamics may alter over time – witness, for example, the dominance of the medical culture in the NHS and the relatively recent rise of the management culture (Bourn and Ezzamel 1986; Harrison and Nutley 1996; Jones and Dewing 1997; Sutherland and Dawson 1998). Thus, some subcultures may share a common orientation and similar espoused values, but there may also be disparate subcultures that clash or maintain an uneasy symbiosis (Martin and Seihl 1983; Degeling *et al.* 1998).

Researchers have adopted two broad frameworks for studying organizational subcultures. The first defines subcultures relative to an organization's overall cultural patterns, especially its dominant values (Martin and Seihl 1983). From this perspective subcultures are classified in terms of whether they support, deny or simply co-exist alongside the values of the dominant culture (see Box 1.8). The second framework acknowledges that subcultures relate to occupational, departmental, ward, speciality, clinical network and other affiliations (Scott *et al.* 2003a). Arguably, these two perspectives need to be synthesized, as elements of both are likely to be found within any large-scale organization. For example, the NHS is a distinctly British institution with a recognizable overall identity and certain apparent core values. Within that overall 'NHS culture', a number

---

Box 1.7   Commonality and difference in organizational cultures

- *Integrated*: Integrated cultures occur when there is broad-based consensus on the values, beliefs and appropriateness of behaviours within the organization. Although often assumed, such integration may exist only in aggregate, or may be more aspirational than realized.
- *Differentiated*: Differentiated cultures occur when multiple groups within an organization possess diverse and often incompatible views and norms. The development of subcultures, misunderstandings and conflicts is then to be expected. The NHS has long existed as a collection of loosely coupled differentiated cultures (medical, nursing, professions allied to medicine, administrative and, more recently, managerial groups).
- *Fragmented*: At the most extreme, differentiated cultures may diverge and fragment to such an extent that cross-organizational consensus and norms are absent. Even within specific groups, differences may be more marked than commonality, and agreements that are seen may be only fleeting and tied to specific issues. Thus the organization may be characterized by shifting alliances and allegiances, considerable uncertainty and ambiguity, and unpredictability.

This typology is *not* intended to suggest that organizations have cultures that are either integrated or differentiated or fragmented. Instead, *each* of these views may be applied to the *same* organization to reveal, rather than hide, an overall lack of coherence.

Source: Adapted and extended from Martin (1992)

---

of distinct subcultures can be discerned whose relationship to the overall organizational culture is hard to disentangle.

Rivalry and competition between groups may appear as a key feature of the overall organizational culture (health care is notoriously tribal in this respect: Harrison *et al.* 1992; Harrison and Nutley 1996). Different subcultures may be more or less malleable (susceptible to managed change of their artefacts, values or beliefs) or may even be avowedly resistant to change (perhaps developing the status of 'counter cultures'). Indeed it is apparent that some organizations function more or less successfully with discordant subcultures, with each subculture being no more than 'loosely coupled' to other subcultures or subsystems (Harrison *et al.* 1992; Harrison

---

Box 1.8   Classification of subcultures

Complex organizations such as hospitals can be characterized as comprising a variety of co-existing subcultures. Three types of subculture can be identified vis-à-vis their organizational functionality:

- *Enhancing cultures*: these represent an organizational enclave in which members hold core values that are more fervent than and amplify the dominant culture. For example special hospital units which constitute centres of excellence.
- *Orthogonal cultures*: an organizational subgroup that tacitly accepts the dominant culture of the organization whilst simultaneously espousing its own professional values. An example in the NHS is clinicians' allegiance to the Royal Colleges.
- *Counter cultures*: an organizational enclave that espouses values that directly challenge the dominant culture. For example, clinical resistance to management diktat, or the new contractual obligations and limitations on clinical freedom wrought by the rise of managed care in the US.

---

and Nutley 1996; Degeling *et al.* 2003). Nonetheless, different subgroups may still share certain key cultural attributes whilst conflicting on others, for example, whilst doctors and managers may differ on many different cultural dimensions (see Box 1.9) they both 'inhabit a shared culture of medical autonomy' (Harrison *et al.* 1989). It remains an open question as to whether it is even desirable that an organization should seek an integrated set of cultural attributes.

ACCOMMODATION ACROSS DIVERGENT SUBCULTURES

Child and Faulkner (1998) developed a useful typology to classify the various approaches to managing cultural diversity. In essence, two fundamental policy choices or possible outcomes in the management of cultural diversity were identified. First is whether one partner's culture should *dominate*, as opposed to striving for a balance of contributions from the contributory cultures. The second choice addresses whether to attempt an *integration* of the partners' cultures (with the aim of deriving synergy from them) *versus* a preference for segregating the cultures within the organization (with the

---

Box 1.9   Managerial and medical cultures: points of divergence

	Managerial	*Medical*
Structure	bureaucratic	collegial
Group loyalty	low	high
Job security	low/medium	high
Disciplinary base	social sciences	natural sciences
Evidence base	case studies on organizations	clinical studies on patients
Focus	patients as groups	patients as individuals
Skills	managerial/human relations	biomedical/technical
Allegiance	organization/corporate goals	patient/professional
Discretion	low – rules/procedures	high – clinical freedom
Success measure	efficiency	effectiveness
Quality emphasis	consumer-rated quality	technical quality
Performance review	public	confidential
Professional status	emerging	established
Social status	medium	high
Public trust	low	high – but vulnerable

Source: Reproduced from Davies *et al.* (2000)

---

aim of avoiding possible conflict and reducing the effort devoted towards cultural management). These policy choices give rise to four possible bases for accommodating cultural diversity: synergy, domination, segregation or breakdown (see Box 1.10). The first three offer a basis for establishing cultural fit, whilst the fourth results in inaction or organizational damage. At different times each of these outcomes has been seen in UK health care (Box 1.10) – although whether these were as the result of deliberate policy choices is doubtful. More considered attempts at cultural transformation will need to address explicitly the importance of managing cultural diversity in order achieve cultural fit.

Box 1.10 The meeting of cultures: achieving a cultural fit

Four possible bases for accommodating cultural diversity within health care organizations can be identified depending on whether there is integration between subgroups and/or domination by one of the subcultures.

Integration between subgroups?

	Yes	*No*
No	**1 Synergy** The objective is to meld both partners' cultures and to achieve the best possible fit between the two. The best elements are combined with the objective of making the whole greater than the sum of its parts. The combination of management and clinical roles by clinical directors is an example of this.	**2 Segregation** Here the aim is to strike an acceptable balance between different subcultures by virtue of maintaining separation rather than seeking integration. In many health systems inter-professional alliances may be seen to be of this type. For example accommodation between the nursing profession and doctors
Yes	**3 Domination** This is based on recognition that integrating subcultures may prove impossible and accepts the right of dominance of one subgroup's culture. Clinicians have traditionally assumed this role and have until recently been largely self-regulating rather than being the subject to external monitoring and assessment.	**4 Breakdown** This occurs when a subgroup seeks domination, integration or mutually acceptable segregation but fails to secure the acquiescence of the other group. For example failed attempts in advanced health systems over many years to usurp the dominance of the medical profession.

(left margin, vertical:) **Domination by one subculture?**

Source: Derived and expanded from a classificatory scheme on strategic alliances developed by Child and Faulkner (1998)

CULTURAL CHANGE

Having discussed the origins and nature of organizational culture, and some of the implications of this metaphor for considering organizations, we now turn to discussions of how culture may change – both through its own dynamic and through planned management action.

Cultural formation and transformation

Although certain cultural traits may endure within an organization, culture is dynamic and shifting, rather than static. It is *dynamic* in that there may be rapid swings in organizational norms (e.g. in response to organizational crises such as funding shortfalls, or manifest clinical errors), and *shifting* in that longer term and more consistent drifts may occur (e.g. the gradual acceptance of an overt management culture in the NHS; the growing recognition of quality failings in the NHS). Newcomers to an organization may bring with them prior expectations about the culture when they join, but culture is also transmitted to new arrivals by established staff, sometimes explicitly but more often implicitly. The organizational culture is shaped and articulated not just by individuals but also by new and old organizational features. The organizational structures, routines, command and control expectations, and operational norms all have influence (Langfield-Smith 1995). Large gaps may develop between overt statements about culture (such as the values espoused in hospital mission statements) and the implicit communication of the same (for example in the ways in which services are managed and delivered). Organizational culture can also be influenced by factors outside of the organization (Langfield-Smith 1995). The strong professional ethic and sense of professional identity seen in the health professions attest to the importance of supra-organizational norms. Public opinion, the media and regulatory frameworks also exert influence (Davies 1999). All these observations have implications for those attempting to manage a cultural shift.

First and second order cultural change

Identifying differences in the *scale and pace* of cultural shifts allows a distinction to be drawn between first order and second order organizational change (Bate 1999). During first order change the objective is to 'do what you do better'. Many commercial organizations have, for example, maintained a competitive advantage by pursuing a policy of 'cultural continuity', capitalizing on the lessons, traditions and working practices that have served the organization well over a period of time. The focus in first order change is on evolutionary growth or quantitative reproduction and repetition (more of the same). In contrast, second order, qualitative growth (something different) is more appropriate if an existing culture has begun to stagnate and a complete overhaul is required. Such second order change is often invoked in response to a growing crisis or deficiency in the existing culture, which cannot be addressed adequately by a change *in* culture but rather demands a fundamental change *of* culture. Thus second order change focuses on instilling *new* behaviours and values throughout the organization, whereas in first order change the emphasis is more on adapting and refining the *extant* culture and traditional modes of working.

Models of cultural change

The relationship between organizational change and culture is intimate: most models of change see some role for the collective assumptions, values and beliefs in attempting to bring about shifts in collective practice (Scott *et al.* 2003c). A diverse range of models for understanding organizational change have been developed, usefully reviewed by Iles and Sutherland (2001). From this diversity it is unsurprising that models of cultural change are also varied, this variation reflecting a lack of theoretical consensus surrounding both definitions of organizational culture (outlined above) and the processes of organizational change. Whereas those viewing culture as an organizational attribute or variable might be more open to the possibilities of managed cultural change than those in the 'culture as metaphor' camp, nonetheless significant divergence remains. For example those conceptualizing culture as shared norms (e.g. Kilmann 1984) can be more optimistic about purposive change than those seeing culture more in terms of deep assumptions (e.g. Lundberg 1985; Schein 1985a, b, 1990) – shared norms may be viewed as being more readily amenable to open identification, challenge and change than deeper assumptions.

Brown (1995) summarized a wide range of models of culture change drawn from the literature. Despite some manifest differences between the models reviewed, they all share some common foci:

- *Crises*: as a trigger for significant organizational change.
- *Leadership*: in detecting the need for change and in shaping that change.

- *Success*: to consolidate the new order and counter natural resistance to change (as one of the functions of organizational culture is to establish and stabilize a way of living, resistance is inherent to any culture change efforts).
- *Relearning and re-education*: as a means of embedding and helping explain the assimilation of new cultures.

As leadership is accorded a central role in many models of cultural change, it is to this issue that we now turn.

Leadership and organizational culture

Leadership has been a prominent theme in the work of many writers on organizational culture (Pettigrew 1979; Smircich and Morgan 1982; Schein 1985b; Kotter and Heskett 1992; Bryman 1996). Indeed, according to Schein (1985b) 'the unique and essential function of leadership is the manipulation of culture'. However, one source of confusion lies in the lack of a clear distinction between leadership and management. Early writers such as Selznick (1957) tried to make a distinction by linking leadership with critical decision making. In the development of this line of thinking, routine decisions are seen as being made by ordinary administrators or managers, whereas strategic concerns – such as an organization's mission, identity and development – are key leadership issues (Zaleznik 1977; Kotter 1990). Thus the essential difference between leadership and management lies in their orientation towards organizational change (Bryman 1996), with leaders engaged in the crucial task of managing the underlying organizational culture. Leaders (usually conflated with 'senior management') were then seen as the most prominent and legitimate vehicle by which to capture the hearts and minds of employees. Notwithstanding this, there has been little real consensus between scholars concerning either the proper definition of leadership or what constitutes an appropriate analysis of its role in achieving significant organizational change.

The leadership literature, separately from that of organizational culture, has developed in a number of phases: the *trait approach*, dominant up to the 1940s; the *style approach*, prevalent from then until the 1960s; the *contingency approach* (1960s to 1980s); and more recently the *'new leadership'* and *'dispersed leadership'* ideas of the past two decades (Bryman 1996).

- *The trait approach*: This approach is based on the belief that leaders are born and not made. It seeks to identify and isolate the essential leadership qualities of those who have achieved positions of power and influence.

- *The style approach*: Although trait research has lingered on, the style approach favours a shift in emphasis away from leadership as personal attribute and towards an understanding of leadership behaviour. Along with this comes a change in focus away from selecting leaders and more on preparing and training those in leadership roles.

- *The contingency approach*: The contingency approach to leadership examines the situational variables that moderate the effectiveness of different types of leadership. This line of thinking is against notions of leadership as an essential quality held by some people and not others, and sees leadership as more than merely a set of practised behaviours.

- *The 'new leadership' approach*: These approaches which emerged in the 1980s used a variety of terms including transformational leadership (Bass 1985), charismatic leadership (Conger 1989), visionary leadership (Sashkin 1988), or just simply 'leadership' (Bennis and Nanus 1985; Kotter 1990). These labels share a common conception of leaders as managers of meaning, as visionaries, and as creators/interpreters of organizational symbols.

- *Dispersed leadership*: In addition to the focus by some 'new leadership' research on heroic individuals at the apex of organizations, researchers have also studied leadership exhibited at various levels in the organization, conceiving the leader as local facilitators who cultivate the group and remove obstacles from its path.

In sum the leadership literature is as diverse and contested as that of culture. However ideas within the 'new leadership' and 'dispersed leadership' paradigms seem best fitted to understanding the cultural change process in health care. In particular, a common distinction between 'transformational' processes (the wholesale renewal of values, assumptions and sense-making in an organization) and 'transactional' processes (day-to-day incremental administration) seems useful in assessing the interactions between organizational culture and key stakeholders (see Table 1.4). That the transformational leadership literature also has significant weaknesses – it has had little to say, for example, about informal leadership processes, has rather ignored contextual constraints on organizations, and has tended to focus on 'successful' organizations, to name but some – can more properly be seen as challenges for the design of future empirical work.

Table 1.4   Transactional and transformational management

	Transactional change	*Transformational change*
Context	Predictability Urgent need for improvement Short-term targets	Uncertainty and flux Fast changing sector Long-term need for growth/innovation
Leadership and senior management team	Planning and monitoring Detailed, hands-on, control Hierarchical command structure	Setting scenarios, intent and direction Creating values/purpose Encouragement/coaching
Navigation and measurement	Dedicated full-time project management Critical path networks Operational/financial targets Micro measures	Change as part of normal responsibilities Co-ordination through communication Balanced score cards Macro measures
Ownership	'Need to know' involvement Following instructions and procedures Top-down messages	Extensive involvement 'Breakthrough' culture Self-initiated change and learning
Enabling	Redesign of organizational structure(s) as lever	Facilitation and knowledge management – people do it for themselves

Source: Adapted from Locock (1999)

Practical ramifications for NHS cultural change

The 'cultural vision' for the National Health Service has undergone significant shifts at important policy junctures (see, for example, Box 1.11). Given that further attempts are to be made at a cultural transformation within health care providers (building on, for example, clinical governance (Donaldson 1998; Scally and Donaldson 1998)), what are the issues that need to be considered? From this reading of the literature, a number of guiding principles can be discerned:

Box 1.11   Changing cultural visions in the NHS

	The vision for the NHS, mid-1980s to mid-1990s (general management and the internal market)	The vision for Labour's 'New NHS', late 1990s (the Third Way)
Macro/system level factors		
Basis of economic relationships:	*Competition (contracts)*	*Co-operation/ partnership (long-term service agreements)*
Governance:	*Market discipline*	*'Third way'*
Key objectives:	*Efficiency*	*Efficiency/equity/ quality*
Rate of change:	*'Big bang'*	*Evolutionary*
Locus of change:	*Top down*	*'Everyone's business'*
Flows of information:	*Confidential/com- mercially sensitive*	*Open/transparent*
Basis of performance assessment:	*Finance/activity/ volume*	*'Balanced scorecard'*
Micro/clinician level factors		
Basis of practice:	*Professional judgement*	*Evidence-based*
Basis of control:	*Mutuality/trust*	*Audit, external verification*
Clinical performance information:	*Confidential*	*Publicly available*
Participation in audit (e.g. confidential enquiries):	*Discretionary*	*Mandatory*
Accountability:	*Largely opaque (professional self- regulation)*	*Transparent: corporate and clinical governance*

Public confidence:	*High*	*Diminished*
Continuing professional development:	*Discretionary*	*Mandatory*
Ethical basis:	*Hippocratic oath/ patient first*	*Corporate objectives*

Source: Reproduced from Davies *et al.* (2000)

- *Wholesale and simultaneous change on all the many different aspects of organizational culture is unfeasible and probably not even desirable.* For example several valuable cultural traits already exist in the NHS on which any new quality strategy can build, most notably a commitment to equity and belief in the founding principles (i.e. a universal, comprehensive service, available to all without regard to ability to pay). More recent helpful values that are beginning to emerge include, for example, the centrality of patient care, a belief in evidence, and a growing willingness to examine safety and quality issues – although these values may be conceptualized rather differently by different professional groups. Thus any strategy for cultural change should be selective, aiming for a balance between continuity (first order change) and wholesale renewal (second order change), identifying those cultural aspects to keep and reinforce, and those which need to be reworked.
- *The nature of the cultural destination for the NHS and other health care organizations is currently far from clearly specified.* Much work remains to be done on defining a vision for a 'transformed NHS' in terms of its cultural assumptions, values and artefacts. Shortell and colleagues (1998) have identified what they termed 'characteristics of the new moral fabric' which may help define some of the future directions (see Table 1.5), and a close reading of official policy documents and accompanying commentaries allows elucidation of other possible aspects of the desired cultural change (Davies *et al.* 2000; Department of Health 2001a) (see also Box 1.11). However, what these shifts mean for day-to-day practice has yet to be properly analysed, assessed and communicated.
- *Cultural change cannot easily be wrought from the top down by simple exhortation.* Successful cultural change strategies need to take into account the needs, fears and motivations of staff at all levels (Beer *et al.* 1990). Further, any attempt to influence culture

Table 1.5 Characteristics of the old and new 'moral fabric' for clinicians (context for culture)

Old expectations	New expectations
Clinician responsible only for individual patient	Clinician responsible for individual patient and populations of patients
Individual clinical responsibility for patient	Team or group, and patient, responsibility
Credibility and trust largely based on professional mystique and prestige	Credibility and trust based on data and documented evidence of effective practice
Profession determines performance and accountability criteria	Profession and others (governments, purchasers, public, community groups, etc.) determine performance and accountability criteria
Clinician accountable to patients and the profession	Clinician accountable to organization and other non-professional agencies
Organizations exist to serve individual clinicians' interests	Organizations exist to serve patient, community and clinician interests

Source: Adapted from Shortell *et al.* (1998)

needs to be part of a much wider assemblage of mutually reinforcing improvement activities (Williams *et al.* 1996). The organizational culture cannot be tackled in isolation from such issues as the organizational structure, financial arrangements, lines of control and accountability, strategy formulation or human resource management initiatives.

- *Observed behavioural changes may not represent real changes in culture*. Simple behavioural changes arising from interventions may not necessarily reflect true cultural change – underlying beliefs, values and assumptions may be largely unaffected. Of course, if these new behaviours do become thoroughly embedded and routinized, then this may, in time, influence deeper cognitive change. Thus, deeper cultural change *may* occur as a result of surface behaviour change, but is not synonymous with such change. One corollary of this is that any culture change strategy might helpfully aim to influence *both* deeper cognitions and surface manifestations.

- *Coherence within the organization may be helpful but may not be sufficient to bring about substantial change.* The influence of outside professional bodies (such as the BMA or the Royal Colleges), specialist societies, patient interest groups and the media may cut across and sometimes work against internal reform efforts. Identifying areas of consensus and consistency in the values espoused by these organizations and attempting limited cultural shifts in these areas may therefore be advantageous.
- *Cultural diversity within the organization needs careful management.* Large and diverse subcultures are known to exist in health care (Degeling *et al.* 1998, 2003). Accommodating these in any new cultural milieu will require careful integration strategies (Child and Faulkner 1998) as well as an appreciation of the potential merits and functionality of such diversity.
- *Leadership has a crucial role to play in cultural change.* Understanding leadership in terms of 'dispersed leadership' provides multiple 'points of entry' for those interested in managing cultural shifts.

CONCLUDING REMARKS

Economic institutions such as culture are important, and underpin a wide range of economic activity. However, although frequently invoked, notions of organizational culture are often under-specified. Unpacking the character of these, and exploring the nature of any linkages between culture(s) and performance, thus remains an important task. This review of the conceptual underpinnings concludes that considerations of organizational culture (and any relationship of this with performance) cannot be made in isolation from two other preoccupations of organizational scholars: the role of leadership and the management of change. This review therefore recaps on current thinking in these areas as a means of providing some structure against which the empirical work could be devised, analysed and interpreted. The next chapter examines the pre-existing evidence base in support of any culture/performance relationship, before exploring the empirical findings emergent from the project.

NOTE

1   Selznick actually used the term *institution* here. However, we have chosen to use the term *mini-society* to preclude confusion with the (albeit related) economic use of the term *institution* introduced earlier.

2

DOES ORGANIZATIONAL CULTURE INFLUENCE HEALTH CARE PERFORMANCE? A REVIEW OF EXISTING EVIDENCE
(with Tim Scott)

INTRODUCTION

The notion that organizational culture can affect health care performance rests upon certain assumptions: that health care organizations, units or work groups have identifiable cultures; that culture is related to performance; that a culture can be altered to impact on performance; and that the intervention will provide a worthwhile return on investment, with benefits outweighing any dysfunctional consequences. Thus, a link between culture-based interventions and improved organizational performance is contingent on a chain of assumptions of uncertain strength or validity. In view of the widespread activity and investment in this area, and prior to developing our own fieldwork, we wanted to know if any reliable evidence could be found to support the contention that aspects of health care organizations' cultures are related in significant ways to aspects of their performance.

RELATING CULTURE AND PERFORMANCE

Much work outside of health care has attempted to make linkages between organizational (or 'corporate') culture and subsequent organizational performance. Several populist texts of the 1980s expounded these links, for example, Peters and Waterman (1982) claimed to have uncovered the corporate cultural characteristics leading to 'excellence'; Ouchi and Wilkins sought to explain links between culture and productivity (Ouchi 1981; Ouchi and Wilkins 1985); and various authors argued for the importance of 'strong cultures' as a way of ensuring high corporate performance (Deal and Kennedy 1982; Denison 1990; Gordon and Di Tomaso 1992). This 'excellence' literature has however not been without its critics (Saffold 1988; Gordon and Di Tomaso 1992; Wilson 1992). These have called attention to the unsubstantiated assumption of a unitary culture that underlies such work, the lack of an operational definition of cultural 'strength', and the weak methodologies employed in the original empirical work (indeed, many of the corporations initially identified as excellent subsequently turned in poor performance). A review of more recent studies came to somewhat more cautious conclusions about any culture–performance relationships (Wilderom *et al.* 2000).

Wilderom and colleagues reviewed ten major quantitative studies (the major empirical/quantitative culture–performance studies to date) in an attempt to substantiate the culture–performance link (Wilderom *et al.* 2000). Nine of these ten studies, carried out in diverse US and European industries, purported to find associations between cultural characteristics (such as strength, consistency or adaptability) and both short- and long-term performance (such as sales, growth or return-on-investment). Yet in collating the evidence, the review's authors drew attention to the diverse methodological difficulties that precluded the drawing of strong conclusions supporting such a link as causal (not least the ambiguity surrounding definitions of both culture and performance). Further, all of the studies included were nomothetic in design, and thus none could shed much light on *how* such associations might be accomplished. Indeed, given the cross-sectional nature of the studies, the data are equally consistent with the hypothesis that performance determines cultural traits rather than vice versa. In addition, the authors raised concerns over publication bias, noting that quantitative studies that find no linkages between culture and performance are less likely to reach major journals. In sum then, the reading of the evidence *outside of health care* highlights some of the difficulties in linking culture to performance and does not reveal a strong empirical base in support of the relationship.

Organizational culture change may also have broader effects than those intended. Unintended, unforeseen (and often unwanted) results could be predicted to occur as culture changes. These may be minor and inconsequential or major and dysfunctional (Martin 1992; Legge 1994; Hawkins 1997). While a range of unintended consequences may be expected to arise from *any* management intervention (e.g. Smith 1995a), those taking place as a result of culture management have been surprisingly little studied. Nonetheless, two significant publications that explored empirically this issue in a series of case studies (Harris and Ogbonna 1998; Harris and Ogbonna 2002) did uncover a range of unintended effects. These included the ritualization and dilution of change, the erosion or selective reinvention of culture by frontline workers, and the appropriation of culture change processes for other purposes. These findings suggest that any examination of culture and performance should broaden its scope, looking beyond positive predicted effects and encompassing an examination of unintended and dysfunctional outcomes.

Thus the evidence base to date linking culture and performance in *non*-health care organizations is suggestive but far from definitive. However, these ideas have now percolated into health care, forming major strands of both policy stipulations and managerial action. This begs critical review. This section therefore retrieves and reviews the major empirical evidence linking organizational culture and performance specifically within health care organizations.

SEARCHING FOR EVIDENCE

The methods of literature search and summary are described in detail elsewhere (Scott *et al.* 2001, 2003d), but in brief we employed a comprehensive electronic search to uncover all the major pieces of empirical work examining a culture–performance link in health care organizations. The initial search strategy was designed with the help of information professionals at the NHS Centre for Reviews and Dissemination, and began by searching the following databases for articles on organizational culture: Medline, Cinahl, King's Fund, Helmis and Dhdata. These databases combine coverage of all the major English language management journals with an emphasis on health services research.

The resulting records were assessed for relevance by two of the research team, and full articles apparently dealing with culture and performance in an empirical manner were retrieved. Bibliographies of these articles were also searched, and the authors of articles and culture measurement tools (Scott *et al.* 2003d) were contacted wherever possible. In addition, as part of the scoping study, we had extensive discussions with around 30 subject area specialists during the two seminars in London (UK) and Berkeley (US). These allowed us to be reasonably confident that we had uncovered all the major empirical studies examining links between organizational culture and health care performance.

From over 1700 bibliographic records initially uncovered and assessed, 69 full articles were retrieved. Of these, ten reported empirical studies of relationships between organizational culture and performance in health care organizations. Only one of these studies was based solely in the UK. One covered hospitals in the UK, Canada and the US; the remaining eight were based in American health care organizations.

REVIEWING AND SYNTHESIS

Standard systematic review methodology, with quantitative aggregation of effects, is impractical and inappropriate when reviewing the linkage between such diverse and contested concepts as 'culture' and 'performance'. There is simply insufficient conceptual or methodological common ground to make true systematic review methods tenable. Instead, we present a qualitative narrative review of studies found after a comprehensive and documented search process.

The aim was to use an examination of published work to advance knowledge in a number of areas. First, we wanted to understand further the nature of organizational culture and its expression within health care organizations. Second, we wished to examine, in all its diversity, the current state of evidence in the health care arena linking cultural aspects to aspects of performance. Third, we were interested in extracting the methodological lessons to inform the development of further empirical work. Thus this review does not attempt to aggregate heterogeneous findings but uses instead a brief narrative on each study (see Table 2.1) followed by some integrating discussion.

The narrative on each study is informed by a number of critical questions: how were both culture and performance conceptualized? To what extent were the culture and performance variables distinct? Was it clear which of these was the dependent and which the independent variable? And finally, if performance *was* reported as being related to culture, what was the nature of any such relationship?

Table 2.1 Studies relating organizational culture and performance

Study	Participants	Context	Culture levels	Culture assessment	Performance indicators	Summary of findings
Jackson 1997 UK Ideographic	Patients and staff of UK hospital outpatient department	Study of the effect of outpatient culture on non-attendance rates	Level 1: behaviour patterns Level 2: attitudes, values and beliefs	Non-participant observation and telephone survey	Number of patients who did not attend appointments	A link between culture and performance (non-attendance rates) is supported. This suggests the importance of examining the mutual production of organizational culture between staff and clients
Argote 1989 USA Nomothetic	Physicians (463) and nurses (278) working in 44 emergency units in US hospitals	Comparative study on relationships between norms and work-unit effectiveness	Level 1: behavioural norms	Normative complementarity (agreement *between* groups) Normative consensus (agreement *within* groups)	Work-unit effectiveness, including: promptness of care, quality of nursing care, quality of medical care	The results tend to support a linkage between culture and performance. Between group norms appear to be more important for high performance than within group norms

Table 2.1 *continued*

Study	Participants	Context	Culture levels	Culture assessment	Performance indicators	Summary of findings
Gerowitz et al. 1996 USA, UK and Canada Nomothetic	Top management teams of 265 hospitals, 120 in the USA, 100 in the UK, and 45 in Canada	Comparative study of top management culture and hospital performance	Level 2: values	Competing Values Framework (Cameron and Freeman 1991)	Employee loyalty and commitment; external stakeholder satisfaction; internal consistency; resource acquisition; and overall adaptability	As hypothesized, the dominant culture of the hospital management team was positively and significantly related to aspects of organizational performance valued in that culture. A contingent link between culture and performance is thus supported
Gerowitz 1998 USA Nomothetic	Top management teams of 120 hospitals in the USA (n=271)	Study assessing the impact of TQM/CQI on culture and performance of top management	Level 2: values	Competing Values Framework (Cameron and Freeman 1991)	Adaptability and global performance measured subjectively by managers	A link between culture and performance is partially supported: culture focus and culture orientation both accounted for significant variations in performance differences. However,

| Nystrom 1993 USA Nomothetic | Senior managers (n=41) and executives (n=36) in 13 US health care organizations | Study of the impact of culture on organizational commitment, job satisfaction, and performance; and examination of the relationship between culture and strategy | Level 1: norms; Level 2: satisfaction, commit-ment, values | Kilmann-Saxton Culture-Gap Survey. Managerial Values Questionnaire. Organizational Commitment Questionnaire. Job Diagnostic Survey (see Nystrom 1993 for these) | Managers' judgements comparing the overall performance of their organization with other organizations producing similar services | A link between culture and performance is claimed but there are significant methodological problems. In particular, many of the performance measures used (job satisfaction, job commitment and perceptions of relative performance) might more appropriately be considered as cultural characteristics |
| | | | | | | use of subjective assessments of performance confuse dependent and independent variables – a serious methodological concern |

Table 2.1 *continued*

Study	Participants	Context	Culture levels	Culture assessment	Performance indicators	Summary of findings
Rizzo *et al.* 1994 USA Nomothetic	235 nursing department staff from 13 units in the US	Analysis of nursing unit culture and work characteristics to inform change in care delivery	Level 1: behaviour patterns	Nursing Unit Cultural Assessment Tool (Coeling and Simms 1993)	Unit skill mix; cost measures; worked hours; quality assurance monitors; documentation of care and discharge planning; patient satisfaction	Only one unit had reached its one-year evaluation mark. It is unclear if a link between culture and performance is supported, or not
Shortell *et al.* 2000 USA Nomothetic	3045 CABG patients from 16 US hospitals	Study to assess the impact of TQM and culture on organizational performance	Level 2: attitudes, beliefs and values	20-item version of the Competing Values Framework (Cameron and Freeman 1991)	Risk-adjusted clinical outcomes, functional health status, patient satisfaction, cost measures	A link between culture and performance is not generally supported. However, the way in which hospitals were selected, and the relatively low power of the study to detect even quite large effects (80% to detect odds ratios of 2 or more for various outcomes) means that this study more properly reflects an absence of evidence

| Shortell et al. 2001 USA Nomothetic | 56 medical groups in the US involving 1797 physician respondents | Cross-sectional study examining the role of market pressures, compensation, and culture | Level 2: attitudes, beliefs and values | 20-item version of the Competing Values Framework (Cameron and Freeman 1991). Patient-centred culture measure (Kralewski et al. 1996) | Evidence-based care management measures derived from medical group key informants | Whilst implementation of evidence-based care was significantly associated with economic incentives such as compensation and the presence of managed care pressures, there was no apparent relationship with culture. The authors suggested this was perhaps because of the amorphous, recent and superficial nature of many US medical groups |

Table 2.1 *continued*

Study	Participants	Context	Culture levels	Culture assessment	Performance indicators	Summary of findings
Zimmerman *et al.* 1993 USA Ideographic and nomothetic	3672 ICU admissions, 316 nurses and 202 physicians	Study to examine organizational practices/culture associated with higher and lower performance in the ICU	Level 1: awards and ceremonies; rituals, learning/ teaching. Level 2: attitudes, beliefs and values	Interviews and direct observations; Organizational Culture Inventory (Cooke and Lafferty 1987)	Ratio of actual/ predicted death rate (effectiveness). Ratio of actual/predicted duration of ICU stay (efficiency).	Some important relationships were identified: superior organizational practices among the ICUs *were* related to a patient-centred culture, strong medical and nursing leadership, effective communication and co-ordination, and open, collaborative approaches to solving problems and managing conflict. However, structural and organizational questionnaires, self-evaluation by staff members, and the research team's implicit judgements following detailed

Study	Sample	Cultural level	Measures	Findings
Zimmerman et al. 1994 USA Ideographic and nomothetic	888 ICU admissions, 70 nurses and 42 physicians	Study to examine structural and organizational characteristics, including culture, at two ICUs with divergent risk-adjusted survival	Level 1: behavioural norms	Creativity, task preferences, communication style and mutual support were measured by an (unnamed) organizational and managerial process questionnaire	on-site analysis all *failed* to distinguish higher and lower performing units. A link between culture and performance outcomes is thus not supported
				Risk-adjusted mortality ratio. Mean actual to mean predicted ICU length of stay ratio. Mean actual to predicted ICU resource utilization ratio. Self-evaluated technical quality of care. On-site investigator ranking	Structural and organizational questionnaires, self-evaluation by staff members, and the research team's implicit judgements following detailed on-site analysis all failed to distinguish higher and lower performing units, A link between culture and performance outcomes is again not supported

THE EVIDENCE UNCOVERED

The ten studies uncovered differed in terms of the types of health care organizations studied, participants included, levels of culture assessed, set of performance measures included and methodologies applied (Table 2.1). This variety should not be surprising as, for example, culture embraces many aspects of organizational life and the performance measures chosen may relate to the goals seen as relevant within participating organizations. Thus the indicators of performance used included indices of service quality in hospitals (Argote 1989), hospital employee loyalty and commitment (Gerowitz *et al.* 1996), and risk-adjusted clinical outcomes for cardiac surgery patients (Shortell *et al.* 2000). Assessment of culture also varied greatly, including both quantitative and qualitative assessments of norms (Argote 1989; Gerowitz *et al.* 1996; Shortell *et al.* 2000) and employee attitude and beliefs (Shortell *et al.* 2000, 2001). One notable feature was the failure of any of the studies to go deeper than observed artefacts (Level 1) or explicit statements of attitudes/beliefs (Level 2) to explore deeper assumptions (Level 3) (Schein 1985a, b).

The studies also varied methodologically, from ideographic (i.e. concerned with the individual, pertaining to unique facts and processes) non-participant observation and depth interviews (Jackson 1997), to large-scale nomothetic (i.e. concerned with the discovery of general laws) statistical analysis (Shortell *et al.* 2000, 2001). Two studies used mixed methodological approaches (Zimmerman *et al.* 1993, 1994).

Of the ten studies, four found some evidence for a link between culture and performance (Argote 1989; Gerowitz *et al.* 1996; Jackson 1997; Gerowitz 1998), four found little evidence for such a link (Zimmerman *et al.* 1993, 1994; Shortell *et al.* 2000, 2001) and two provided unclear findings due to significant methodological issues (Nystrom 1993; Rizzo *et al.* 1994). An outline of each of these studies is given in Table 2.1; a fuller narrative review of each follows.

Culture and paediatric outpatient non-attendance in the UK

The only study conducted solely in the UK (Jackson 1997) was also the only one to adopt an entirely idiographic approach to examining the relationship between culture and performance. (Two other studies that supplemented their nomothetic stance with some idiographic data collection are discussed later – Zimmerman *et al.* 1993, 1994).

Non-participant observations of a hospital paediatric outpatient department were used to view the processes and attitudes of patients and staff during a typical outpatient session (Jackson 1997). Such observations were supplemented with a telephone survey of patients/parents of patients who did not attend for their hospital appointment. This telephone survey also included interviews with a similar number of matched controls. The author asserted that her findings suggested that a relationship between the outpatient department's culture and patients' attendance did exist – but that the precise nature of this relationship was unclear.

The first key issue highlighted by this study was the potential interplay between the organization's culture and patient behaviour. For example, if reception staff do not attend promptly to patients, this is likely to affect patients' attitudes and may influence subsequent decisions to default on attendance. High levels of non-attendance may, in turn, influence staff attitudes and behaviour toward patients. Recognition of this interplay suggests that examinations of culture in health care may need to be broadened to capture such recursive relationships.

Second, while the design of this study prevents any conclusions from being drawn on our central question, it does serve to highlight a serious conceptual/methodological problem alluded to above – that of distinguishing between culture and performance. What the investigator actually observes in the study are two aspects of process performance (how staff enact their roles and patients enact theirs) together with a performance outcome (the did-not-attend rate). Yet the behaviour of both staff and patients, and the high default rate in turn, could all be construed as artefacts of the organization's culture. Such ambiguity complicates the search for a link between culture and performance, as such a link is premised on the belief that these concepts are formally and substantively distinguishable from one another.

Cultural norms and unit effectiveness in US hospital emergency units

The relationship between cultural norms and unit effectiveness was tested in 44 hospital emergency units in the US (Argote 1989). Two dimensions of culture were analysed: *normative complementarity* (the amount of agreement *between* professional groups about the norms governing their relationships), and *normative consensus* (the amount of agreement existing *within* a group about their norms). Organizational effectiveness measures included three dimensions:

promptness of care, quality of nursing care and quality of medical care.

Regression analysis showed that normative complementarity and normative consensus explained a significant amount of variance in each of the effectiveness indicators. As normative complementarity and/or normative consensus increased, the promptness and quality of care also increased. The effect sizes were larger and statistically significant for the measures of between-group agreement (complementarity), but smaller and not significant for the within-group measures (consensus).

This study therefore suggests that *agreement about norms between groups* is positively and significantly associated with the effectiveness of emergency units, whereas the relationship between performance and normative agreement *within* professional groups is weaker and less clear. Such findings tend to agree with earlier work (Krackhardt and Stern 1988) which found that organizations with strong between-group ties were more effective than organizations with strong within-group ties, in crisis situations. As crises are everyday occurrences in emergency units, and therefore not crises in the usual sense, these findings indicate that a similar relation between inter-group normative agreement and performance may also exist in non-critical situations.

This study suggests that groups sharing a high common understanding of emergency situations work together better than do groups with a lower common understanding of those situations. Yet, in similar situations, the level of agreement between individuals within the groups does not make any significant difference. This is a potentially important finding, as it suggests that there may be something about the primary–secondary group relationship that differs from the individual–primary group relationship. It also supports the view that groups and individuals are different units of analysis, with consequent methodological implications for culture and/or performance assessment.

Top management culture and hospital performance in the UK, US and Canada

Gerowitz and colleagues (1996) examined the role of top management team culture in 265 hospitals located in Canada (45 hospitals), the UK (100 hospitals) and the USA (120 hospitals). The competing values framework (Cameron and Freeman 1991; Gillies *et al.* 1992) was used to identify clan, open, hierarchical and rational cultures (see Chapter 5 for more detail on these culture types). Five measures of performance were used: (1) employee loyalty, (2) external stakeholder satisfaction, (3) internal consistency, (4) external resource acquisition, and (5) overall adaptability. Three empirical questions were then addressed:

1 Whether hospital management teams in the USA, Canada and the UK have different management cultures given the differences in their political economies.
2 Whether management culture was associated with differences in performance.
3 Whether using culture types derived from the competing values framework was a fruitful research avenue in seeking to explore variations in performance.

The paper concluded that the empirical findings supported each of these propositions. First, there was evidence that the political economy influenced the distribution of culture types: hospital management teams in the UK were more frequently clan and hierarchical cultures; hospital teams in the USA were more frequently rational and open cultures; and hospital management teams in Canada were more frequently clan and rational cultures.

Second, the data provided significant support to the overall hypothesis that culture is linked to performance. A key finding was that the dominant culture of the hospital management team was positively and significantly related to organizational performance in the case of clan, open and rational cultures, *but only in the performance domain valued by that culture.* For example, hospitals with dominant clan cultures performed significantly above average on measures of employee loyalty and commitment; those with dominant open cultures performed better on measures of external stakeholder satisfaction; and those with dominant hierarchical cultures were significantly different in the internal consistency domain from those that exhibited clan, rational and open cultures. Thus these findings also support the final proposition, providing some empirical legitimacy for the use of cultural typologies in examining variations in hospital performance.

This study again highlights the interdependency of culture and performance – a recurrent feature in most of the studies reviewed. That certain culture types perform better than others against the measures that they value highly, suggests that they are successful in expressing and realizing those values. But this also underlines the relativity of performance measures and begs an important question:

who wants performance? Or alternatively *performance according to whom?*

TQM, culture and performance of top management in US hospitals

In 1998 Gerowitz published another study, to assess the impact of TQM/CQI interventions on the culture and performance of top management teams in 120 hospitals in the USA (Gerowitz 1998). The competing values framework was again used to assess culture type, and the performance indicators measured were adaptability and overall performance as gauged subjectively by managers.

The analysis found no significant associations between performance and TQM/CQI initiation. However, significant relationships between performance and culture were uncovered. Externally focused cultures (open and rational cultures) were associated with high performance, and internally focused cultures (clans and hierarchies) were associated with low performance. However, no significant association was found between performance and culture *orientation* (mechanistic hierarchical and rational cultures versus relational clan and open types).

Along with its exclusive attention to US hospitals, this study also uncouples the performance criteria from culture type, thereby losing some of the subtlety of the earlier comparative study. Whereas the first study used a variety of different measures of performance, the second simply used managers' subjective assessments of overall performance – again confusing dependent and independent variables. Thus this study was unable to examine the more subtle hypotheses that specific cultures are related to specific aspects of performance, and could not clarify the nature of any culture/performance relationship.

Culture, organizational commitment, job satisfaction and performance in US hospitals

Nystrom (1993) similarly focused on higher management echelons in a study of the impact of task norms and pragmatic values on employee outcomes, including organizational commitment, job satisfaction and performance. Performance was measured by asking managers to compare the overall performance of their organization with other organizations producing similar products or services. The organizations were also classified by 'strategic type' (Miles and Snow 1978: prospectors, analysers, defenders and reactors). Senior managers (n=41) and executive secretaries (n=36) in 13 health care organizations in the USA were included.

The results show that culture does appear to affect employee outcomes and performance. Job satisfaction and organizational commitment both correlated significantly with task norms and pragmatic values (job satisfaction was also correlated significantly with organizational commitment, as has been found elsewhere – Alpander 1990). The results also showed that organizational cultures differ for health care organizations pursuing alternative strategies. The distribution of task-norm scores for managers who see their organizations pursuing a consistent strategy (prospectors, analysers or defenders) is compared with the distribution of task-norm scores for managers who see their organization operating with an inconsistent strategy (reactors). The organizations with an inconsistent strategy tended to exhibit weaker norms and weaker values than did organizations pursuing any of the three consistent strategies.

According to the author, these results show that a stronger culture is more effective than a weaker one, but this conclusion does not directly follow from the data. The results show that when senior managers are strongly committed to their jobs and perceive the organization's strategy to be coherent, they are more committed to the organization and get greater job satisfaction. These results tell us little, however, about the relationship between an organization's culture and any external (objective?) measures of performance.

Nursing culture and performance in the USA

An analysis of nursing culture assessed 235 nursing department staff in 13 units as a precursor to changing their care delivery model (Rizzo *et al.* 1994). Nursing unit culture was measured by the Nursing Unit Cultural Assessment Tool (NUCAT-2 – Coeling and Simms 1993). Performance was measured in terms of unit skill-mix, cost, worked hours per patient day, quality assurance, documentation of care planning and discharge, and patient satisfaction. The premature report of this study prevents any conclusions being drawn: only one unit had reached its one-year evaluation stage. Further, the results reported (focusing on a reduction in professional nursing staff, cost savings and increased working hours) suggest a thinly veiled cost-cutting exercise rather than a concerted research effort to examine relationships between culture and performance.

Culture and performance in cardiac bypass surgery in the USA

A more substantial and rigorous study, by Shortell and colleagues (2000), assessed the impact of TQM and organizational culture on performance in terms of a wide range of outcomes for 3045 patients undergoing coronary artery bypass grafts (CABG). As in the papers by Gerowitz *et al.* (1996) and Gerowitz (1998) described previously, culture was again measured by the competing values framework (Cameron and Freeman 1991). Unusually however, this study defined performance directly in terms of patient outcomes: using risk-adjusted clinical outcomes including mortality and length of hospital stay, functional health status and patient satisfaction. Here then we see a more concerted effort to maintain a distinction between the concept of culture and that of performance.

The results from this study show that although a 2- to 4-fold difference in all major clinical CABG care endpoints was observed among the 16 hospitals, little of this variation was associated with TQM or organizational culture in any systematic way. For example patients receiving CABG from hospitals with high TQM scores were more satisfied with their nursing care but were more likely to have lengths of stay greater than ten days; a supportive group culture was associated with shorter post-operative intubation times but longer operating room times; and a supportive group culture was also associated with higher patient physical and mental functional health status scores six months after CABG. Overall, the study provides only weak and inconsistent evidence of associations between culture and performance.

Culture and the implementation of evidence-based care management in the USA

A second study by Shortell and colleagues (2001) again used the competing values framework, as well as a separate physician-specific 'patient centred culture measure' (Kralewski *et al.* 1996) in a bid to explain the implementation of evidence-based care management in US physician organizations. The study found that while implementation of evidence-based care was significantly associated with economic incentives such as compensation and the presence of managed care pressures, there was no apparent relationship with culture. The authors explained the apparent absence of any effect by noting that physician organizations in the USA were more collections of physicians joined together under a legal umbrella, rather than coherent organizations with much that was shared.

Culture and Intensive Care Unit (ICU) performance in the USA

Zimmerman and colleagues (1993) also failed to find evidence for a link between culture and performance in a study involving 3672 ICU admissions, 316 nurses and 202 physicians in 9 ICUs. Culture was assessed using a combination of interviews, direct observations and questionnaires, including the Organizational Culture Inventory (Cooke and Lafferty 1987). Effectiveness was measured by the ratio of actual/predicted hospital death rate, and efficiency was measured by the ratio of actual/predicted length of ICU stay.

On the basis of each unit's risk-adjusted mortality rates, nine out of 42 ICUs were selected for intensive on-site analysis by investigators blinded to the actual mortality rates. Using semi-structured interviews, examination of physical artefacts and observation, each investigator developed a summary report which was shared and discussed by study members, and combined with all summary reports to create a composite report for each unit. In this way a listing of the 'best' and 'worst' cultures, leadership, co-ordination, communication and problem-solving practices was developed, along with the potential effect on ICU performance. Each investigator also rated the nine ICUs (best to worst) according to anticipated final risk-adjusted mortality ranking.

The results of the on-site assessments indicated that superior organizational practices amongst the ICUs were related to a patient-centred culture, strong medical and nursing leadership, effective communication and co-ordination, and open, collaborative approaches to solving problems and managing conflict. However, the on-site case studies failed to identify accurately those units with significantly better or worse performance in terms of risk-adjusted survival. This failure may be due to a mismatch between the subjectively based on-site investigations and the objective assessment of actual risk-adjusted mortality. Interestingly, however, Zimmerman *et al.* conclude that the cause of the problem lay in their performance criteria: 'we believe the inaccuracy of the rankings was related to . . . the absence of an objective value-free process for arriving at criteria on which to evaluate performance' (Zimmerman *et al.* 1993).

The final health care organizational study of culture and performance, is a follow-up to the above study (Zimmerman *et al.* 1994). This later study focused on two ICUs with marked differences in risk-adjusted survival: the actual hospital death rate was 21 percent for Unit One and 6 percent for Unit Two. When adjusted for case-mix, the standardized mortality rate at Unit One was significantly worse (1.21; p<0.05) and at Unit Two significantly better (0.76; p<0.05) than that across all 42 ICU study sites. However, the findings of this more detailed study of two units do not differ from those of the earlier study. Neither the global judgements of the on-site investigators, nor self-evaluation by unit physicians and nurses, accurately ranked Units One and Two according to risk-adjusted mortality. In addition, on-site observations and questionnaire data regarding culture, leadership, co-ordination, communication, and problem-solving/conflict management did not clearly distinguish between higher and lower performing units.

MAKING SENSE OF THIS EVIDENCE

Cultural comparisons (across countries or corporations) are not especially new: the intimacy of the relationships between attitudes/beliefs and economic structures/performance has long been seen as being bound up with national or group cultures (Hofstede 1980; Fukuyama 1995). The organizational culture perspective extends this work to help explain performance differences between different organizations (Deal and Kennedy 1992; Hofstede 1994; Brown 1995; Davies *et al.* 2000). Recent and related work by West (2002) suggests that culture-related factors such as the human resource policies in hospitals, especially those regarding staff appraisal, may have important implications for realized performance, even in areas such as risk-adjusted mortality (West 2002). Similarly, previous work largely outside of health care contains individual studies claiming to have uncovered important culture/performance relationships. More systematic reviews, however, are rather more sceptical of the eviden-tial base for such claims (Wilderom *et al.* 2000). This is also the key message from this review of studies in the health care arena: we found some, problematic but nonetheless supportive, evidence for the relationship between organizational culture and health care per-formance, but the evidence base is not extensive. It is also clear that any relationship between culture and performance is unlikely to be simple: such relationships are far more likely to be multiple, complex, contingent and dynamic.

Our review of empirical work examining linkages between organizational culture and health care performance found some, problematic but supportive, evidence for the relationship. Four of the ten studies reviewed in detail claimed to have uncovered evidence for the hypothesis, and whereas the other studies failed to find clear relationships, none found much evidence against. Most convincing of the evidence that encourages further study in this area was that provided by the initial work by Gerowitz *et al.* (1996). This study found three important things. First, that health care organizations do differ in measurable ways in their dominant cultural orientation; second, that this cultural orientation is associated with various aspects of performance; and third, that if we want to understand relationships between culture and performance we should explore aspects of performance that are valued in the dominant culture. It is this final point that is most instructive in questioning the idea that relationships between culture and performance will be simple: they are far more likely to be multiple, complex and contingent.

The failure of six of the ten studies to uncover much evidence linking culture to performance might more properly be seen as an absence of evidence rather than evidence of absence (Altman and Bland 1995), not least because of the formidable methodological difficulties in this area. Although no formal comparative assessment of methodological quality was undertaken (and, given the method-ological diversity, such an approach would have been difficult), all of the studies used predominantly cross-sectional designs and would have benefited from longitudinal aspects to their approach. Further, the sampling of units in which to examine the culture–performance link was often far from ideal, and sample sizes often led to a lack of power to detect appreciable effects. In addition, there remain many concerns over how culture and performance are assessed and related.

Assessments of culture

Most of the studies focused on culture at level one (patterns of behaviour) and level two (espoused attitudes, values and beliefs). That none addressed level three (assumptions) is both a shortcoming and a testimony to the difficulties of so doing. However, as Schein has identified (Schein 1985a, b), we can begin to uncover implicit assumptions by looking for discrepancies between espoused values and actual practice. This in turn draws attention to the predomin-ance of quantitative methods used in the studies: addressing discrep-ancies between espoused views and observed behaviours will require far greater utilization of qualitative methods.

Four of the studies (Gerowitz *et al.* 1996; Gerowitz 1998; Shortell *et al.* 2000, 2001) used a typology approach to assessing culture rather than continuous variables. In each case, the approach chosen was based on the competing values framework. This approach has a strong provenance in social theory and organization studies and allowed more nuanced investigations: not, *does culture affect performance?* but, *which cultures are related to which aspects of performance?* Qualitative assessment of cultures was deployed in three studies (Zimmerman *et al.* 1993, 1994; Jackson 1997). The latter two studies by Zimmerman and colleagues failed to identify correlations between these qualitative assessments and performance, but the authors attributed this more to the difficulties of identifying appropriate performance indicators rather than as signs that the culture assessments were deficient. Qualitative culture assessments would seem to be capable of offering rich descriptions of great potential value, for example in providing better underpinning to behaviourally-based economic models (Fuchs 2000).

Assessments of performance

Defining performance presents further problems, as there exists, for any organization, a range of possible measures. This is true especially of health care, with measures of clinical process, health outcomes, access, finance, productivity and employee variables all offering some potential (Mannion and Goddard 2002). In addition, different channels of communication may convey different performance information, for example the apparently 'hard' information contained in league tables may differ from the 'softer' intelligence circulating around informal networks (Goddard *et al.* 1999, 2000).

The essential ambiguity of performance arises from three main senses of the nature of 'performance': performance as *enacted behaviour*, relating to socio-technical processes of care; performance measured in terms of *endpoints or outcomes*; and performance as a *dramatic event*. Each of these meanings tends to invoke the other two, as befits the nature of signification in general. A surgical procedure, for instance, implies both a technical performance and a desired outcome, as well as entailing aspects of dramatic production and presentation (for example from whose perspective is success or failure determined?) A consultant's ward round is a ceremonial vehicle for demonstrating important social and technical competencies, including diagnostic skill, communication, therapeutic knowledge and learning. Finally, performance data – whether relating to waiting times, medical errors or comparative data on mortality – of necessity imply a series of socio-technical processes behind the bald statistics. The use of such data calls for skills in the timing and presentation to target audiences, often with the aim of persuading or otherwise influencing behaviour. Armed with this understanding of the complexity of 'performance' we approached the empirical literature with open minds, prepared to classify specific definitions of performance or revise the framework as necessary.

The studies examined a wide variety of measures of performance. This highlights the difficulty at the heart of performance assessment in health care, which may also help to explain why its relationship with organizational culture is so hard to determine: there is almost as much dispute regarding how to define performance in health care as there is about defining culture (Smith 1995b, 2000). Although frequently presented as a hard-nosed, bottom-line concept, performance is, in practice, almost as nebulous, elusive and complex as culture. Thus performance may be seen to be less a singular, objective phenomenon and more as something multiple and contested, with understandings that are both negotiated and socially mediated. Further, as there is no consensus – or even clearly hypothesized suggestions – as to which outcomes should be affected by which cultures, we should not be surprised that many studies fail to find any clear effects.

A related issue concerns the degree of separation between independent and dependent variables in some of the studies. It is questionable, for example, to assess the effect of espoused values on employee loyalty and commitment (Gerowitz et al. 1996), when such measures of performance are indeed values themselves. Likewise, can subjective judgements of managers on their own organization's performance (Gerowitz 1998) be viewed as external to that organization's culture? At one extreme, organizational culture as 'the way things are done around here' (Davies et al. 2000; Davies 2002) sounds suspiciously like a definition of realized performance. Thus there is a danger of confusing cause and effect, and so clouding rather than illuminating any culture–performance link.

A further difficulty lies in disentangling the direction of any causality between performance and culture. Although most of the attention has focused on how culture affects performance, it is equally plausible that certain cultures emerge from high-performing organizations. That is, that performance drives culture. More likely still is that culture and performance are reciprocal, recursive and mutually reinforcing – in a manner that is thoroughly dependent on wider context and influences.

CONCLUDING REMARKS

Whether we term it a culture or an institution, it seems certain that the local social systems at the heart of health services are both impacted by and set limits on structural and procedural change (Le Grand *et al.* 1998; Davies 2002). Dealing with these cultural issues is a key challenge in managing change in any organization, and shaping culture is a (perhaps *the*) core component of leadership (Smircich and Morgan 1982; Schein 1985b; Kotter and Heskett 1992; Bryman 1996). Thus the proposition that organizational culture (however defined) and health care performance (in all its variety) are linked has enduring intuitive appeal – yet it is currently supported by little firm evidence. Considerable conceptual and empirical work remains to be done to provide better substantiated articulation of what these links might be – and what their implications are for health care policy and management. Crucially, it is not enough to know whether culture is linked to performance – we also need to discover how and why it is linked (e.g. technically, psychologically, linguistically, politically). For only then can we decide if policies, strategies and interventions are appropriate, and think through how they could be better designed. The following chapters present freshly gathered evidence linking culture and performance in the NHS that addresses both these concerns: *whether* there is a link, and *how* such links might be expressed and mediated.

3

CULTURE AND PERFORMANCE IN ACUTE HOSPITAL TRUSTS: INTEGRATION AND SYNTHESIS OF CASE STUDY EVIDENCE

INTRODUCTION

In this chapter we draw on rich qualitative case study evidence to explore the established organizational practices, styles of management and shared working assumptions that taken together form the basis of organizational cultures in English acute hospital trusts. Our findings are based on an integration and synthesis of evidence drawn from across a purposeful sample of six case studies. Condensed narrative accounts of each supporting case study follow in Chapter 4.

To focus the discussion we present the case study evidence arranged around some key current policy concerns pertinent to the design of performance management and clinical governance arrangements in the NHS:

- the key cultural characteristics of apparently high and low performing hospital trusts;
- senior management visions for planned culture change within their organization;
- the levers and facilitators that are thought to foster culture change in hospital trusts;
- the key barriers and inhibitors to beneficial culture change in these organizations;

- the unintended and dysfunctional consequences of culture change programmes in hospital trusts.

However, before reporting the empirical findings, we first outline the nature of the case study evidence and detail the sampling strategy used to select the participating organizations.

CASE STUDY EVIDENCE

We used a purposeful sampling strategy to generate six case studies comprising organizations at either end of the performance spectrum. Two high performing acute hospital trusts (three star rated) and four low performing (zero or one star rated) acute hospital trusts (see Table 3.1). The subsequent analysis involved triangulation of supporting data derived from semi-structured interviews with key staff and evidence obtained from a review of internal reports and external documentation. This has been analysed and assembled into a detailed narrative for each case study site (reported later in Chapter 4), with each narrative retaining its own integrity for the purposes of description, analysis and theory development. Further details of the sampling strategy and methods of data gathering, and data analysis are contained in Appendix 1.

Table 3.1 Background characteristics of the six hospital trusts

Hospital trust	A	B	C	D	E	F
Measured performance	Low	Low	Low	Low	High	High
Hospital type	District general	District general (merged)	District general	Teaching	District general	District general
Location	Town	City	Town	City	City	Town
Income (£million)	Less than 100	Greater than 100	Less than 100	Greater than 100	Greater than 100	Less than 100
Number of beds	Under 1000	Under 1000	Under 500	Under 1000	Under 1000	Under 500

INSIGHTS CONTRIBUTED BY INDIVIDUAL CASE STUDIES

The rich experience intrinsic to each individual case study contributed unique and compelling insights into how the complex inter-linkages between organizational culture and organizational performance are mediated by particular management practices and institutional arrangements. Therefore, as a prelude to a discussion of the themes that can be drawn from across the trusts we first of all push to the fore two of the key issues arising from the individual case studies: first, the key role of leadership; and second, the important cultural issues that arise from trust mergers. Subsequent to this, we *draw across* all six case study sites to analyse the culture/performance patterns in hospital trusts.

Leadership (based on the case study of Trust A)

The case study of Trust A (see Chapter 4, pp. 91–103) provides a powerful account of the importance of senior leadership culture in both enabling and disabling the wider organizational culture. As outlined in Chapter 1 the unique and essential function of leadership is the manipulations of culture (Schein 1985b) and recent government policy documents have emphasized the need to unlock the potential for leadership distributed throughout the NHS workforce as a key driver for continuously improving the performance of health care organizations.

Analysis of Trust A contributes valuable insight into the role of leadership in shaping the culture(s) and performance of hospital trusts. Indeed, the quality and nature of the senior management leadership in Trust A was reported to be the dominant influence on the organization's culture and performance. The previous chief executive (a new chief executive had taken over six months prior to the study) was viewed as a very charismatic and dynamic leader who inspired immense personal loyalty amongst an inner core of senior mangers. Indeed, the previous culture of the organization appeared in many ways to be similar to the 'club' culture identified in the Kennedy Report as pertaining to Bristol Royal Infirmary.

In 'club cultures' (Handy 1988) the organization functions as a form of spider's web, with power residing in the centre surrounded by ever widening circles of intimates and influence. The closer individuals are to the 'spider' the more influence they have, and the organization functions as a club or as an extension of the leader's personality.

The danger here lies in the dominance of the character of the central leader. Without a spider the web is dead. If the leader is weak, corrupt, inept or picks the wrong people the organization is also weak corrupt and badly staffed, and finding a new leader becomes critical (Handy 1988). The chief executive of Trust A was reported to have nurtured a senior management team that was largely self-regarding and focused on its own group maintenance needs rather than the wider interests of the organization or its patients. The senior management team was described as being disconnected from the wider organization and lines of accountability were opaque. Organizational rewards were said to be based on patronage (determined by loyalty and personal access to the chief executive) rather than any objective measures of performance.

In seeking to enhance their own national profiles, insufficient attention was paid by the chief executive and the senior management team to developing robust internal performance management processes. Managers outside the inner circle had little input to strategic decision making and this was said to explain why many calamitous and inappropriate decisions were made. Indeed a 'climate of fear' was said to pervade the trust, where staff felt frightened to challenge the chief executive or report mistakes for fear of reprisals. Those who did challenge decisions were 'seconded' to other organizations or otherwise excluded. The lack of attention to performance management issues remained largely a hidden matter, until a critical external report highlighted the weak clinical governance arrangements at the trust.

Staff outside the inner circle welcomed the external scrutiny and the additional leverage this created for changing processes at the trust. Soon after the report was published the chief executive left of his own accord. The new chief executive at the trust adopted a more transactional approach to managing the trust and was focused on developing robust systems for monitoring and improving the trusts performance. He was also reported to have adopted a more inclusive and participatory management style. Staff reported that the organization appeared less cliquey and middle managers now contributed more to the development of policy. The change of chief executive in Trust A thus appears to have influenced the wider culture of the trust, particularly the orientation of the organization towards meeting national performance targets. This case study, therefore, demonstrates the reach and impact of senior management team culture across a broad spectrum of organizational performance.

Cultural integration after trust mergers (based on the case study of Trust B)

The case study of Trust B (see Chapter 4, pp. 104–17) provides significant insights into the difficulties of merging cultures following the merging of organizations. Since 1997, more than a hundred mergers of NHS trusts have taken place, including horizontal mergers of acute hospitals, mental health trusts and community health service trusts (Fulop *et al.* 2002). One of the key aims attached to mergers are the economic gains associated with economies of scale and scope as well as the rationalization of over capacity. The case study of Trust B sheds light on the role of culture in facilitating (and inhibiting) the formation of new organizational identities through a merger policy.

Many of the performance difficulties of Trust B were reported to be rooted in the merger. The two merged organizations were reported to have had very different management styles, formal structures and patterns of working. A residue of these differences appeared to survive the merger and served to stifle collaborative working between the two main hospital sites. An 'us and them' culture had developed and there was considerable animosity between staff at all levels across the sites. This impacted deleteriously on the trust's performance. For example, trust-wide performance management arrangements were compromised, as patient administration systems across the sites did 'not communicate with each other'. There were also inherited differences in approaches towards corporate governance across the sites. One of the merged trusts had an established clinical directorate structure with considerable devolution of responsibility to individual teams; in contrast the other trust was viewed as more centralist with relatively few devolved powers. Because of this difference this hospital site was viewed as being slower to modernize its working practices and was not seen as being fully committed to implementing the new corporate agenda.

The new chief executive at the trust was aware of the serious performance difficulties consequent on the cultural differences across the trust. Concerted efforts were being made to diminish cultural differences and a raft of measures were introduced to improve communication and facilitate joint working across the trust. This case study therefore alerts us to the importance of cultural factors, values and entrenched modes of working that may have a profound influence on negating many of the expected gains from radical structural changes to organizations.

DIVERGENCE IN THE CULTURES OF 'HIGH' AND 'LOW' PERFORMING ACUTE TRUSTS

Beyond their value as individual case studies with many insights for policy and management (narratives for each case study follow in Chapter 4), we integrated across these cases to develop broader arguments as to the nature of the culture/performance link. This identified a range of cultural characteristics of hospital trusts that appeared to be linked in some way to their measured and unmeasured performance. Here we focus on the main points of divergence between the culture(s) of apparently high and apparently low performing organizations. The key cultural differences we found between high and low performing organizations are summarized in Table 3.2. It should be noted that this table serves merely as an organizing framework for summarizing our findings. Whilst we believe that these points of departure are generalizable across the six case studies we would emphasize that there is a patterning of experience that is unique to each organization and that the cultural profile of individual trusts do not necessarily fit neatly into this template. To enrich the description we also provide a brief case study of a high performing trust (Box 3.1) and a low performing trust (Box 3.2) to illustrate how the complex linkages between culture and performance play out in organizations at either extremes of the performance spectrum. Fuller accounts of each case study follow in Chapter 4 (see pp. 91–158).

The key points of divergence identified in Table 3.2 can be grouped under four broad headings, each of which is discussed subsequently:

- leadership and management orientation;
- accountability and information systems;
- human resources policies;
- relationships within the local health economy.

Leadership and management orientation

As discussed in Chapter 1, styles of leadership have been proposed as a key intervening factor between an organization's culture and its performance. Given this, we were interested in exploring the relationship between the dominant styles of leadership in each trust, the influence of this on its overall managerial orientation and how these two factors combined to influence organizational performance.

Table 3.2 Key points of divergence in the cultures of apparently high and apparently low performing hospital trusts

Cultural characteristics	High performing trusts	Low performing trusts
Chief executive	Apollo*	Zeus*
Leadership style	Transactional	Charismatic
Management integration	Fully integrated	Cabalesque/clique
Management orientation	Corporate	Pro-professional
Senior management preoccupation	Meeting national performance agenda	Own group maintenance needs
Senior management team turnover	Low	High
Middle management	Strong, empowered	Under-developed, emasculated
Accountability	Clear	Opaque
Rewards	Performance related	Patronage
Information systems	Highly developed	Under-developed
Performance management	High priority	Low priority (financial)
Recruitment policies	Staff to fit culture	Undiscriminating
Local health economy engagement	Proactive	Reactive
Taboos	Not hitting targets	Challenging senior management

* Handy (1988) likens some leaders to Zeus (principal god of the Greek pantheon, prone to personal and capricious interventions, and from whom subordinates seek patronage), while others are likened to Apollo (god of harmony, rules and order; believer in logic and rationality, formal communication and established systems).

Our case studies suggest a strong relationship between trust leadership and performance. The two high performing trusts (E and F, see pp. 138–58) were both characterized by top down 'command and control' styles of leadership. In both of these trusts there was a long tradition of strong directional leadership from the centre with the senior management team setting clear and explicit performance objectives for the organization and establishing robust internal performance management and monitoring arrangements to support these aims. The chief executives of these two organizations were highly committed to continuously improving the measured perform-

Box 3.1   Case study synopsis of Trust A

The trust was classified as low performing (awarded zero or one star) in the performance ratings. There have been several recent changes at a senior management level, including the recent appointment of a new chief executive. Staff reported that the culture of the old regime was very different from the culture of the senior management team in post at the study. The previous chief executive was viewed as a charismatic and dynamic leader who was capable of inspiring immense loyalty amongst an inner circle of senior managers. However, there was a feeling that the core team was disconnected from the rest of the organization and that members pursued their own group maintenance needs rather than policies that would benefit the trust as a whole. In focusing on external issues and seeking to enhance their own national profiles, insufficient attention was directed at developing robust systems and processes, especially clinical information systems. The trust had a very flat management structure, with a short scalar chain of command and a slim tier of disempowered middle management. Lines of accountability were opaque with responsibility for patient care fragmented across many clinical directorates. The organization was described as pro-professional rather than bureaucratic with a few senior clinicians exerting a disproportionate influence on trust policy. Managers outside the inner circle had little input to corporate policy and many believed that this was a major cause of the trust's problems. Staff talked of a climate of fear hanging over the trust in which staff were frightened to challenge senior management decisions or report clinical errors or near misses for fear of reprisals. Challenging core executive decisions was considered taboo. Little constructive learning was said to have taken place in this environment. Relationships with other organizations in the local health economy were said to be poor and this impacted deleteriously on the trust's performance. There were also concerns that the trust had misrepresented its financial and waiting list figures.

The new chief executive viewed culture change as a key element in the trust's strategy for improving performance. He was viewed as more transactional and more internally focused than the previous chief executive. However, he was also viewed as cultivating a more inclusive and participatory approach to managing the trust. There was a strong feeling that culture change should retain the best elements of the previous regime (dynamism, creativity and innovation) and augment these positive characteristics with better information systems and more robust systems of performance management. There was considerable effort devoted to nurturing a learning culture within the trust in which staff felt safe to report clinical incidents and near misses. Specific barriers to implementing culture change were identified, and centred on finding sufficient time and space given the pressure to hit national targets and the fact that staff from the previous regime retained positions of power within the trust. Although the new chief executive had been in post only a few months (and therefore subject to a honeymoon effect) there was a general feeling that significant shifts in culture had already been achieved. Senior management was perceived as less cliquey and the blame culture appeared to be lifting, as evidenced by a large increase in reported clinical incidents.

ance of their organization, and had established organization-wide structures and systems capable of delivering the external performance management agenda. Both trusts were characterized by a 'can do' culture and the most heinous cultural taboo was identified as not meeting national performance targets. Using Handy's culture typology, these organizations may be characterized as having a *'role culture'* with an Apollo-like leader who values rules and standardized processes which are enshrined into formal systems and procedures (Handy 1988).

Although both high performing trusts had a long history of strong 'top down' style of leadership, it was clear that the limits of this approach were by now being appreciated. There were a range of recent initiatives in both organizations to devolve power and responsibility down to individual directorates and nurture a more participatory and decentralized style of management. In Trust E, a key driver behind devolution was the publication of an external report. This had identified problems around adopting a purely top down approach to performance management, in particular the lack of ownership amongst some staff groups in strategic decision making. However, the implementation of a more decentralized approach to running the organization was still in its infancy and there was clearly a divergence of opinion over the feasibility and desirability of relinquishing central control. In Trust F decentralization was more developed, and individual clinical directorates had considerable discretion over the use of resources. This was feasible because of the existence of very robust performance management architecture, especially the highly developed information systems to monitor financial and clinical performance.

Both of these apparently high performing organizations were also characterized by stable senior management teams, who were reported to have good relationships amongst members of the team and with

Box 3.2 Case study synopsis of Trust E

The trust was awarded three stars in the performance ratings and is noted for its strong performance driven culture. The chief executive has been in post for many years and other key staff have long established positions. The dominant style of leadership and managerial orientation was described as directive and transactional with a focus on meeting external performance targets, although there were signs that this was slowly evolving into more devolved and participatory styles of management. It was widely acknowledged that the senior management team were very well connected into the wider organization and the trust had placed considerable resources into establishing a strong tier of middle management (business managers) who were able to develop robust monitoring and accountability systems that were geared up to deliver the external performance management agenda.

The trust was characterized by a strong 'can do' culture with the ultimate taboo described as not meeting external performance targets. Considerable emphasis was placed on recruiting staff whose personalities and skills fitted the high performance culture of the organization. Attention was also focused on promoting a corporate ethos among clinicians, and other professional groups through a range of human resources initiatives, including specialized training and staff development programmes. The trust has strong and clear lines of accountability with each member of the senior management team having well defined sphere of responsibility. The trust was reported to have a good relationship with other organizations in the local health economy and had adopted a very proactive approach in developing joint working and co-operative action, especially in those areas that impacted on waiting lists and re-admission rates.

However, staff did report that the strong performance management culture of the organization sometimes caused problems that were not picked up by the national performance indicators or formal assessments by external agencies. For example, the emphasis on meeting national performance targets was reported to have distorted some clinical priorities and on occasions militated against the provision of high quality patient care. In addition, the very high performance expectations placed on staff at all levels of the hierarchy was said to generate a very heavy workload and in some cases cause excessive stress and anxiety amongst managers and frontline staff charged with delivering ongoing improvements in quality/performance.

the wider organization, particularly the senior consultants. Indeed, there had been a concerted effort in both trusts to develop a more corporate ethos amongst the senior clinical staff through training and staff development initiatives. There had also been some attempt to align internal rewards to performance outcomes, particularly to performance on the national performance indicators.

In contrast, in the four low performing organizations, the previous senior management regimes (all 'under-performing' trusts had had new senior management teams installed over recent years) were characterized by leaders, in particular chief executives, who although viewed as charismatic individuals were generally regarded as lacking the transactional skills required to develop and maintain robust systems of performance management. It was often suggested across these trusts that meeting the external performance targets (apart from financial recovery plans) was not a key priority for some senior staff. Indeed all the 'under performing' trusts had a history of serious financial problems and management effort was focused on achieving a financial balance rather than on meeting waiting list targets or developing robust clinical governance arrangements.

Many of the previous senior management regimes at the low performing trusts were described as being remote and disconnected from day-to-day issues in the wider organization. Terms such as 'cabal', 'clique' and 'inner circle' were widely used in these organizations to describe the virtual sequestration and sometimes self-regarding nature of the senior management teams. In low performing organizations, loyalty to the leadership group was the dominating cultural trait, with 'whistle-blowing' or questioning of senior management decisions considered the ultimate taboo. In Trust A for example, those staff displaying disloyalty to the core executive team, and in particular the chief executive, were 'dealt' with in a variety of ways. One of the most frequently cited sanctions was to remove 'troublesome' people by 'seconding' them to another organization. Here secondment served the major *symbolic* function of relaying a clear message to staff that disloyalty to the senior management team would not be tolerated. It was reported in turn that loyalty was often rewarded with a range of 'prizes', including promotion and scope to gain career-wise by developing national profiles. There are therefore clear parallels with Handy's notion of a 'power' culture in relation to previous senior management teams of low performing trusts. They had contained a Zeus-like leader, capable of inspiring intense loyalty amongst an inner circle of senior staff where 'doing the right thing' was viewed as supporting and protecting the leader rather than serving the needs of the wider staff group, users or external stakeholders.

Senior management teams in the 'under-performing' hospital trusts appeared to be preoccupied with their 'group maintenance needs'. Thus, for example, in Trust A and Trust D (see pp. 91–103 and 129–38), the previous senior management regimes were widely perceived as primarily concerned with their own advancement within the NHS rather than the interests of the trust as a whole. In focusing their energies on cultivating their career advancement through concentrating on establishing high national profiles, it was reported that the chief executive and key members of the senior management team had 'taken their eyes off the ball' internally and had failed to establish internal procedures and systems capable of delivering the external performance management agenda.

The 'low' performing trusts were also characterized by 'pro-professional' cultures where a few senior consultants who were part of the inner circle seemed able to exert an undue influence over their trust's sense of direction and internal priorities. It was suggested that the powerful influence of the medical staff group diverted the trust's attention towards meeting their own clinical needs and priorities, at the expense of meeting the external performance targets. This was especially true in Trust D where many clinicians had international profiles and felt confident about influencing and challenging the corporate agenda.

'Low' performing trusts were generally characterized by an underdeveloped and disempowered tier of middle management. This was reported to be in part due to a lack of resources available for training and staff development but was also attributed to the typical 'cabal' style of management where key decision making was divorced from the practical concerns and financial constraints of the wider organization. This, it was reported, often had a deleterious impact on trust performance as decisions were sometimes taken, such as the development of a new clinical service, without establishing a strong business case and working through the financial repercussions for other services and departments. In addition, the lack of a strong tier of middle management served as an obstacle to the practical implementation policies determined by the centre, as there was little managerial input into ensuring that high level aspirations were driven through and delivered on the ground. It also militated against further devolution of power within the organizations because management lacked the reporting and enforcement arrangements required to support enhanced devolution and autonomy.

Accountability and information systems

We uncovered striking differences between the formal accountability structures and supporting information systems across the high and low performing trusts.

The two 'high' performing trusts were both characterized by clear and largely unequivocal lines of upward accountability. The centre determined the performance targets and held directorates and staff accountable for meeting these targets (especially when they covered areas included in external performance monitoring). Each of the senior board members had well defined spheres of responsibility and formal reporting arrangements. Both trusts had placed a priority on the development of sophisticated information systems to support the needs of performance management. Both trusts adopted a proactive approach to developing information databases for performance management. For example, Trust E tried to anticipate those areas of performance that might be subject to external performance monitoring in the future, and then monitored these internally using 'shadow' performance systems. This allowed the trust to develop timely information in these areas, flagging up any potential operational problems in meeting potential future indicators.

In contrast, low performing organizations were generally characterized by confused and fragmented systems of accountability. In part such fragmentation was sometimes a legacy of recent mergers (e.g. in Trust B). However, under the previous regimes, clinical directorates had generally been allowed a high degree of freedom and autonomy to manage their own affairs. The general approach that prevailed across the low performing trusts was that clinical performance was a professional rather than managerial concern, and senior managers only intervened in exceptional circumstances. Management theorists have termed such organizations as 'professional bureaucracies' (Mintzberg 1983) where much of the power is concentrated among professional workers and the role of management is to co-ordinate and loosely steer the organization. One outcome of this approach was that there had been little investment in information systems to support clinical governance, which made it difficult to hold clinicians to account for their performance. The severe financial difficulties these trusts faced, and the limited resources available for investment in information technology, exacerbated this situation.

Human resources policy

As highlighted in Chapter 1 recent research has suggested that human resources policies regarding the management of people working in acute trusts, and in particular the quality of appraisal systems, may have a significant influence on clinical outcomes (West 2002).

In our study there appeared to be some key differences between the human resources policies of high and low performing trusts. The two high performing trusts appeared to place considerable emphasis on developing and harnessing the potential of staff to deliver the external performance improvement agenda. These organizations also placed a high priority on recruiting and retaining staff who displayed a high commitment to following the corporate rather than professional agenda. It was reported by senior staff that they had often decided not to recruit in a specific speciality if they believed applicants did not display attitudes congruent with the performance ethos of the organization. These trusts also placed a great deal of emphasis on training and educating clinicians so that they were 'encultured' into pursuing the corporate agenda rather than their narrow professional interests. Thus in these two organizations there were planned efforts to mould the values and behaviour of key staff and the important role of the human resources function was reflected in the high profile of the human resources directors and their representation on the trust board.

In contrast, human resource policies seemed to have been ignored or were underdeveloped by previous management regimes of the low performing trusts. In these organizations financial matters had traditionally taken priority because of pressing needs to meet financial improvement targets and consequently resources were diverted away from 'soft' performance issues such as staff development and retraining programmes.

External relationships

Current NHS policy emphasizes a 'whole economy' perspective to delivering the desired changes in quality and performance (Department of Health 2000b). There is also a growing realization amongst health professionals of all occupational groups that little can be achieved to address public health needs by individual organizations. Thus trans-organizational leadership in health care is becoming the new norm, meaning that effective leaders of organizational change must act in concert with leaders in other health and social care organizations whose active collaboration and co-operation are essential to achieving real improvements in the health of local populations. We found some differences in approaches towards partnership and collaboration with key external stakeholders between high and low performing trusts. The two high performing trusts were both characterized as adopting a very proactive approach towards helping to manage the local health economy. These trusts had close working relationships with key external stakeholders and local health influencing organizations. Indeed it was readily recognized that meeting the governments performance targets, especially those around waiting times and re-admission rates depended crucially on adopting a whole-systems approach to managing the local health economy.

In contrast, the apparently poorly performing trusts were generally characterized by a history of poor relationships with other key stakeholders and organizations within the local health economy. Indeed in some trusts (e.g. Trust A and C (see pp. 91–103 and 118–29)) there appears to have been personal antagonism between the trusts' previous chief executive and key local stakeholders. These poor relationships were held responsible for the trusts' poor performance in some areas (such as high re-admission rates and 'bed-blocking'), and it was believed required a co-ordinated effort amongst local organizations to tackle these problems adequately.

In all the trusts there appeared to be a high degree of uncertainty over the inter-organizational dynamics of the local health economy, particularly given the nascent nature of primary care trusts and strategic health authorities, and there was concern over the potential impact of these new organizations on changing the existing balance of power and accountabilities between local health agencies.

IMPLEMENTING CULTURE CHANGE IN ACUTE HOSPITAL TRUSTS

The latest NHS reforms are based on the premise that a major cultural transformation of the organization must be secured alongside structural and procedural change to deliver desired improvements in quality and performance. In this section we set out in broad terms the culture change policies employed by the six trusts, and focus on four key policy areas pertinent to their change management agenda:

- their visions for culture change, especially around clinical governance;

- the levers and facilitators used to implement culture change;
- the barriers and inhibitors to virtuous culture change;
- the unintended and dysfunctional side effects of culture change.

Visions for culture change

From the interviews with key senior managers and a review of internal documentation it was clear that culture change was a clear priority across all six trusts. Thus, for example, the new chief executive of one trust identified culture change as a key requirement for improving the performance of the organization:

> There is a complex interaction between structure and culture. The Trust needs to change its culture, by building on what works well and addressing what does not work. The culture could be changed without altering the structure but the structure does act as an obstacle to cultural change. The danger that the organisation focuses on structural rather than cultural change must be avoided.
>
> (Extracted from an internal document)

In the low performing trusts, the emphasis focused on instilling *new* behaviours and values throughout the organization, whereas in the high performance trusts the focus was more on adapting and refining the *extant* culture and traditional modes of working. Differences in the scale and pace of change between high and low performing trusts aligns closely with the distinction drawn between first order change (high performing trusts) and second order organizational change (low performing trusts) as set out by Bate (1999) and discussed in Chapter 1.

The targets for culture change across the hospital trusts centred on the following areas:

- *Patient focus*: In all the trusts it was reported that the key focus of culture change policies was the need to instil new values, beliefs and working relationships to support the modernization of services around the needs of patients. In particular, it was recognized that facilitating the involvement of patients (and their carers) in every aspect of improving the quality of services would require radical shifts in entrenched professional practices that had been affirmed in the NHS over 50 years.
- *Corporacy*: A key concern was to nurture an allegiance or 'buy in' of staff to the corporate agenda rather than the parochial con-

cerns of individual service departments. Of particular concern were the problems around the strong allegiance of clinical staff to their professional bodies, including the Royal Colleges, rather than the trust. It was clear that the two high performing organizations had explicitly addressed these issues by attempting to engender a strong corporate spirit amongst the various professional groups. In contrast, the low performing organizations had only recently begun to tackle this cultural issue.

- *No blame*: There were concerted attempts across all the trusts to develop a 'no blame' culture in which staff felt safe and confident to report clinical errors and adverse incidents. In the low performing trusts the emphasis was more on establishing the channels for reporting these issues, whereas in the high performing trusts, where such channels of communication were more firmly established, the focus was on trying to shift the cultural constraints to reporting. In particular it was reported that the performance ethos of these organizations sometimes worked against the open reporting of under performance and clinical errors.

- *Team-working*: Establishing multi-professional team-working was a concern of all the trusts. However, in general, the low performing trusts, because of their strong pro-professional ethos, were finding this harder to achieve than the high performing trusts with their more corporate philosophy. Those trusts with fewer clinical directorates also reported that team-working arrangements were working better because of fewer difficulties in co-ordinating across service boundaries.

- *Control and accountability*: In the low performing trusts a key priority focus of the new senior management teams was on the establishment of strong lines of accountability to facilitate control by the centre. This required a shift in the values of key individual staff who had enjoyed considerable autonomy to manage their own affairs under the previous management regimes. These trusts were characterized by having historically weak accountability structures and monitoring arrangements and it was believed that before additional power and responsibility was devolved to frontline staff it was important to establish robust systems for reporting performance to the centre. The two high performing trusts already had well-established reporting arrangements and were beginning to experiment with devolving more power, resources and responsibility to frontline staff.

Levers and facilitators of culture change

Although all organizational cultures are constantly in flux, their *purposeful* management and manipulation to serve wider organizational ends is a difficult and uncertain business. Our case studies identified a range of levers used by trusts to try to enact culture change:

- *Training and education initiatives*: A range of training and staff development programmes were used in the trusts to help instil new values and working patterns amongst staff. These were provided 'in-house' by some organizations, but were more usually supplied by external organizations such as the Modernisation Agency or private management consultants that had been briefed in relation to the corporate values of the organization. The two high performing trusts had well-established induction programmes for new staff to (attempt to) 'socialize' them into the high performance ethos and 'can do' mentality of the organization.

- *External assessments*: The publication of external evaluation and the NHS star ratings were cited as important catalysts for change, especially in the low performing trusts. For example, it was widely reported that the very critical external report on Trust A (see p. 91) had effectively led to the downfall of the previous regime and had provided a disfranchised staff with a very welcome channel for airing their dissatisfaction. (Such external judgements do not, however, have wholly positive effects.)

- *External organizations*: the Modernisation Agency, the Commission for Health Improvement (CHI, now the Commission for Healthcare Audit and Inspection (CHAI)) and other NHS support organizations such as the Clinical Governance Support Team were often credited with providing the knowledge and expertise required to re-design services around the needs of patients. However, some staff in high performing trusts were aggrieved that these agencies were focused on low performing organizations and had had little input into redesigning their services.

- *Raising the status of nurses*: In some trusts (e.g. D and E) there had been concerted attempts to raise the profile and standing of nurses in the organization. One of the reported objectives behind this was to challenge the traditional dominance of the medical consultants within the organization. Another objective was to break down the traditional deference between nurses and doctors in such a way that nurses and allied professional groups would not feel intimidated when reporting untoward clinical incidents and errors by doctors.

- *Reaction to critical incidents*: It was felt important that the actions of the senior management team in how they treated individuals in relation to specific events (e.g. a person reporting a clinical error or 'whistle-blowing' on financial malpractice) sent a strong signal to the rest of the organization and would influence future behaviour. So in all of the trusts there was increased concern not only to deal with staff in a transparent and fair manner but also to communicate that this had happened to the rest of the organization.

Across the trusts it was recognized that culture management was an important driver for organizational improvement. Although most trusts did not have a stated policy in relation to 'culture change' it was apparent that many policies and programmes within these organizations could be construed as such. The high performing trusts had traditionally focused on this area of activity, whereas the low performing trusts were just starting to get to grips with culture change issues.

Barriers to culture change

Culture change initiatives, such as those identified above, may not always proceed unhindered and therefore a key determinant as to the success or otherwise of a culture change programme may depend on the extent to which barriers to change are surmounted. Across the trusts, managers identified a range of organizational impediments that served to block or attenuate planned efforts at culture change:

- *Vestiges of the old culture*: in some of the apparently under-performing trusts it was reported that efforts at culture change had been stifled because key staff from the previous management regime still held positions of power within the trust. These staff were viewed as an obstacle to redesigning services and nurturing new values and working practices because they represented a strong symbolic link to the past.
- *Lack of resources*: implementing culture change strategies (e.g. staff training and development) requires funding and it was recognized across the trusts that this was a 'soft' target that was readily cut back or sidelined when there were pressures to meet financial targets or channel resources into meeting national initiatives such as waiting times targets.
- *Influence of professional bodies*: across the trusts it was recognized that professional organizations, in particular the Royal Colleges

through their training and accreditation procedures, exerted a formative and continuing influence over the socialization of staff into particular belief systems and modes of working. These professional values were sometimes at odds with the corporate agendas of trusts and served to inhibit modernization processes around the development of multi-professional working arrangements.

- *Government policy*: the influence of wider government policy was viewed as inhibiting the adoption of new cultural values within the organization. For example the government's approach to 'naming and shaming' poorly performing hospital trusts was believed to be entirely inimical to attempts by the acute trusts to nurture a 'no-blame' culture where staff would feel comfortable reporting errors and incidents. The government was also sometimes criticized for 'demonizing' managers for all the ills of the service.

Dysfunctional consequences

In addition to driving beneficial outcomes, culture change policies adopted by the trusts were also reported to have inadvertently induced a range of unintended and dysfunctional consequences for organizations and staff:

- *Tunnel vision*: it was reported that the cultural shift towards meeting the external performance agenda had focused attention on areas of performance that were measured to the exclusion of other important but unmeasured areas. Many clinicians reported that their clinical priorities had been altered to meet short-term waiting targets. For example in Trust F (see p. 149) it was reported that the 13-week target for children's services had forced the trust to concentrate on children referred to it by doctors rather than other professionals, even though the clinical needs of the patients may be very similar.
- *Bullying and intimidation*: the pressures to meet the performance targets was reported to have led to the bullying, intimidation and harassment of staff in some of the apparently under-performing trusts. Given that we largely interviewed senior and middle managers it is not clear whether or to what extent this situation applied to staff lower down the hierarchy. In Trust B (see p. 104), for example, there was a strong feeling that the emphasis on delivering measurable improvements in performance in order to 'turnaround' the organization had contributed to a 'culture of

bullying' in which staff were 'shouted and screamed at' and were threatened with the prospect that 'heads would roll and desks would be cleared' if the national performance targets were not met.

- *Erosion of public trust*: the star rating system may also inadvertently contribute to eroding public trust in health care providers. The case study of Trust B shows clearly how public confidence in the trust had been damaged by the publication of (and hostile press reaction to) a poor star rating classification. It also reveals the extent of the pressures that health professionals labour under in trying to cope with the loss of public confidence in the services that they provide. The diminution in trust consequent on the star rating system is exacerbated by the fact that trust is an asymmetrical commodity which may take many years to establish but can be eroded very easily (Mannion and Davies 2001, 2002; Davies and Mannion 2000). Therefore, even if an acute provider moves from a low to a high star rating it does not necessarily follow that public confidence will be so easily restored. Just as importantly, it also does not necessarily follow that the poor morale amongst staff will improve immediately. Indeed, much intrinsic motivation may have been sacrificed in the process, which may be lost for ever, with management subsequently having to resort to costly extrinsic incentives to drive future performance improvements.

- *Ghettoization*: it was reported that because of its impact on the reputation of acute trusts, the star rating was having a differential impact on the abilities of trusts to attract and retain high quality staff. Whereas all trusts experienced difficulties recruiting staff in some clinical specialities it was clear that the low performing trusts were reporting more serious problems. Staff attributed this in part due to the fact that a high performance rating was attractive in that it signalled to potential recruits the impression that the trust was a good organization to work for. In contrast, low performing trusts reported that a poor star rating contributed to their problems as many health professionals would be reluctant to join an organization that had been publicly classified as under-performing.

- *Insensitivity*: it was reported that the star rating system was too blunt a classificatory device for capturing the complexity of health care performance. In particular there was a strong view across the trusts that all these organizations possessed uneven pockets of good and poor performance that were not accurately reflected in the star ratings because these focused mainly on the delivery of managerial targets. For example, whereas Trust D (see p. 129) was classified as under-performing on the star rating system, it was also rated as one of the highest performing trusts in the country on the Dr Foster league table because of its relative weighting of clinical outcome measures. This, it was reported, caused confusion for staff and the public when judging the performance of the organization. Thus there were concerns that some organizations were being unfairly labelled as under performing (Type I error) or potentially more seriously, that some organizations classified as performing to a high standard were in fact under-performing in areas not included in the star ratings (Type II error). This situation was exacerbated by the fact that external intervention (e.g. by the Modernisation Agency) was often only triggered by a low star rating.

CONCLUDING REMARKS

These six acute trust case studies reveal a strong focus within these organizations on improving health care performance by attending to organizational culture. A wide range of values and behaviours were targeted using diverse levers. That culture and performance are linked in acute trusts, and that the purposive management of culture in attempting to improve performance is widespread, are both greatly substantiated by these studies. However, whether such strategies will prove successful in the medium to longer term remains unanswered (to assess this would require protracted longitudinal study). Nonetheless, intensive case analysis such as this is able to provide a range of insights into the interactions between the external policy environment, senior management team leadership, organizational culture and delivered performance. In the following chapter we present condensed narrative accounts of each supporting case study.

4

CULTURE AND PERFORMANCE IN ENGLISH ACUTE HOSPITAL TRUSTS: CONDENSED CASE STUDY NARRATIVES

(with Alison Powell)

INTRODUCTION

In this chapter we provide condensed narratives of the individual case studies, which taken together form the basis of the integrative analysis presented in Chapter 3. As each case study retains its own validity for theoretical development and generalization, one of our aims is to push to the fore any unique patterning of events or idiosyncratic cultural traits peculiar to each setting. In the narratives we make extensive use of verbatim quotations to drive the discussion. We believe that giving voice to hospital staff in this way not only adds a more authentic and human dimension to the descriptions but also grounds the interpretation within the inter-subjective social reality as perceived and constructed by actors in particular organizational settings.

Data collection in each case study (detailed in Appendix 1) comprised in-depth semi-structured interviews with key managers and a review of relevant internal reports and external documentation. The evidence from both these sources was combined to build a rich understanding of the relationship between culture and performance in each organization. It should be noted that our findings are based on the perceptions and subjective experience of key individuals. Therefore each narrative is drawn from an amalgamation of the reported subjective perceptions, and thus is potentially open to rival interpretations. In order to improve the validity of the study, where possible we cross-referenced accounts between individuals and triangulated the evidence emanating from different data sources. We attempted to reduce the potential for researcher bias by ensuring that at each stage at least two researchers analysed the data and collaborated in the development of coding categories and emergent themes. We also audited the various sources of data in order to search for negative or 'disconfirming' evidence that appeared to contradict or was inconsistent with the emerging analysis. Although we have sought to adhere to the conventional tenets of good qualitative research (which are themselves contested), we make no purist claims of objectivity. Indeed we fully endorse (and celebrate) the reflexive position and acknowledge that our prior assumptions, and methods of research and analysis will necessarily have exerted an influence over our findings.

Given the highly sensitive nature of the material we have sought to protect the anonymity of individuals and their organizations. The trusts where the case studies took place are described in only very perfunctory terms to guard against identification. Quotes are attributed only and as much as is necessary for their interpretation whilst still protecting anonymity. In presenting the hospital case studies, for example, we only attribute verbatim quotes to an organization (Trusts A–F) and do not link speech to specific job titles (with the occasional exception of attributions to trust chief executives where this was important for interpretation). Throughout the case study accounts we resort to use of male personal pronouns to further protect anonymity (a large majority of the interviewees were indeed male, nonetheless we offer due apologies to those legitimately offended by gendered language).

Each case study narrative follows its own logical structure but is ordered broadly as follows. First, limited background and contextual information is provided on each organization. There then follows a discussion of the four performance related cultural characteristics that formed the basis of *a priori* investigation and analysis: leadership style and management orientation; accountability and use of information; learning and reflexive practice; and the quality of external relationships. Any unanticipated issues that *emerged* from the case study analysis are then discussed. For example in all the low performing organizations these include details of the culture change strategies implemented by the new chief executive (all of the low performing organizations had recently appointed a new chief executive). Similarly, an emergent theme common to some, but not all, the case studies was the potential for purposeful culture change policies to induce a range of unintended and dysfunctional consequences for organizations and staff.

TRUST A   HOUSE OF CARDS

Introduction

Trust A is a large district general hospital. It was assessed as low performing (classified as zero or one star) in the NHS performance ratings. There have been several recent changes at senior management level, including the appointment of a new chief executive. As all of the performance measures reported for the trust (including its star rating) were the responsibility of the previous chief executive we first focus on the culture of the trust under this chief executive. We then we explore the culture change strategies being implemented under the new chief executive.

Leadership style and management orientation

Our interviewees described many of the trust's performance problems as originating from the style of management pursued by the tight-knit core executive team (comprising the chief executive, chairman, director of finance, director of human resources and a few senior clinicians). The senior management team was dominated by the very strong personality of the chief executive. He was described as a very charismatic figure and a *transformational leader* who inspired immense personal loyalty and support among an 'inner circle' of senior managers. Many of the core executive team had worked together elsewhere and it was believed that had engendered a strong bond of loyalty to the team rather than the wider organization:

> [What was the style of leadership?] I would say charismatic. The previous Chief Executive was a very high profile person who had a regime, which was based on

personal relationships. So he dealt in a very effective and amusing way with individuals and it was always seen to be slightly disloyal to maybe say that things weren't running very well or that people were waiting in A&E for beds.

The previous Chief Executive slowly but surely drafted in a team around himself of people he had worked with previously at [name of another trust] – people he rated as friends in the NHS – and he created a very, very, tight team of people.

There was an 'in-crowd' and an 'out crowd'. A lot of the older consultants felt marginalized under the last chief executive. He surrounded himself by people of his own generation and outlook.

Staff reported that under the previous management team a general climate of fear pervaded the organization. Indeed, senior managers (those outside the inner circle) reported that they were often frightened to challenge core executive decisions:

You would never take the cabal on. You wouldn't ever tackle them head on . . . So you carried out orders you were given. You tried to put a professional slant on things but there was no point going into battle because they were so strong. I think people were very pleased when they saw the house of cards fall.

It was quite a threatening culture in the fact that there was a very strong core executive management team which was very inspirational, very strong and a very strong synergy about it.

Those who committed the ultimate taboo of challenging core executive policy or 'annoying' the chief executive were dealt with in a variety of ways. One of the most frequently cited sanctions mentioned was to remove 'troublesome' people from the organization by seconding them to another trust. Whereas secondments are generally viewed as a positive development opportunity, staff at the trust reported that the practice of secondment served a major *symbolic* function within the organization in that it relayed a clear message to all staff that 'disloyalty' to the senior management team, and in particular, the chief executive, would not be tolerated. It was also reported that loyalty was sometimes rewarded with increased status within the organization and other forms of patronage. Indeed many staff felt that rewards within the organization, especially at a senior management team level were not related closely to an individual's performance:

> [The Chief Executive] would say 'You're seconded' and secondment was shorthand for being moved out of the trust all together. At one point we had about 27 people seconded – but in the official report it was only 10.

> The vast majority of the trust were very frightened and if they stepped out of line they'd be sent off on secondment. And secondment got to be a really dirty word in this trust. I remember [one of the core executive team] saying to me. You don't sack senior managers at the [name of trust] you just put them on secondment.

It appears that the middle tier of management at Trust A effectively became disempowered under the previous regime as they had little input into the design of corporate policy or the development of business cases for expansion. Some attributed the trust's poor performance, especially its financial predicament, to the lack of wider managerial input into key decisions affecting the organization:

> From a finance and activity point of view you had decisions made by the executive management team, which often went against the view of the wider management team. So for example a consultant had gone to the general management team and said look we need another consultant here. But the general

management team were very clear. 'No we can't afford it'. So on many occasions consultants then went to the executive team when our decision was overridden. The general management team, including myself felt very disempowered.

There's a very real feeling amongst middle managers in the organization, be they in directorates or other functions, that the executive team didn't want to know problems, and there was a view that people who brought problems would be scape-goated, or cold-shouldered or ignored.

[The chief executive's] great trait was doing deals with the boys behind the back of the bicycle sheds, through the back door. And that really alienated a lot of general managers. We had a massive turnover of general managers at one point.

Some staff, however, did identify areas where there had been a positive relationship between the style of leadership of the previous regime and the performance of the trust. Indeed, a few stated said that they had originally been attracted to the trust because they had been attracted by the charismatic personality of the chief executive and the high national profile of individual members of the senior management team. There was also a feeling by many staff that the NHS 'star' performance rating system failed to reflect a balanced assessment of the trust's overall performance, in particular the focus on managerial performance in the ratings was thought to ignore many aspects of innovative clinical work that was performed at the trust.

Although I've been quite negative in some of the things I've been saying . . . I joined this trust because I wanted to work with [name of person in senior executive team] because he was a national figure, somebody I'd read about . . . If you were 'in' it was a lot of fun . . . I enjoyed the fruits of quite a lot of that, although I was never completely in, I made sure I never was, and I could see the dysfunctionality of what was going on.

There are lots of people who are working extremely hard in this trust, and there are some fantastic things going on at an individual level in different clinical areas but they are not reflected in external measures and some of these things are extremely difficult to measure.

Accountability and use of information

Lines of accountability within Trust A were reported to be opaque, confused and fragmented. Information systems, particularly those around monitoring clinical performance and quality were seriously under-developed. This situation was exacerbated by the division of the trust into a large number of separate clinical directorates which created problems in terms of co-ordinating patient care and served to promote 'in-fighting and turf wars' between directorates. Many managers were often unsure about their areas of responsibility and to whom they were accountable. Although budgets were controlled centrally, considerable discretion over clinical matters was devolved to the directorate level. Given the trust's poor financial status the focus on performance review in the directorates had been around finance rather than clinical quality and there appears to have been little corporate ownership for the quality of clinical care provided by the organization. Responsibility for clinical matters was reported to be an entirely clinical concern. Indeed, the organization was described as being 'pro-professional and anti-bureaucratic'.

[The previous chief executive] used to call us a flat management structure. What it meant was if you took a difficult area like medicine for example, by splitting it up and giving a lot of freedom to key figures, those people were kept happy and developed their service but the big picture was lost.

It was essentially a medically dominated culture, by a few key clinicians having direct access to the executive directors and missing out on the middle tier of management who felt alienated.

Another part of the control was establishing very small directorates. So people weren't quite sure of what other people were doing, but a lot of these consultants were given additional responsibility to be clinical directors, it was like being part of the chief executive's club and enjoying the benefits of being part of that club.

Many staff reported that key decisions made by the core executive team were often not recorded in minutes or reports and that this 'oral accountability' reduced the transparency of decision making within the organization. Given the lack of formal information on performance, essential information was transmitted via a variety of informal channels, 'trusted' colleagues and a diverse range of soft intelligence networks:

Very little was written down, so there's very little documentary evidence of agreements being in place. They were more than capable of writing things down but they chose to work in a different way.

[The chief executive] didn't do much formal information, very little attention to detail was paid.

Very little was put in writing. A lot of conversations where somebody asked someone to do something wouldn't necessarily put it in writing.

Internal–external focus of senior management

It was widely expressed that the core executive team at Trust A had focused primarily on furthering its own group maintenance needs and the career aggrandisement of its members, sometimes at the expense of the best interests of the wider organization. The main focus of the core executive team was on external opportunities rather than internal matters. Many of the senior management team served on national committees or carried out other external work. There was a strong feeling that the focus on the national agenda diverted managerial attention away from the development of strong internal processes within the trust. Indeed some staff expressed incredulity that the organization was 'touted' by senior staff as a 'beacon of excellence' within the NHS, when in fact they were aware of serious deficiencies in the management of the trust:

> [It was externally rather than internally focused?] Yeah that was definitely the case. And the NHS has a problem because what do you do when you've done six or seven years of being a trust chief executive. How do you plan your career. One of the options is to start doing some stuff outside the organization but there needs to be an explicit agreement about how you backfill behind that to ensure that the operational issues within the trusts are still addressed.

> There was much that we were seen to be at the cutting edge of service development, but all the basics and underpinnings were not focused on. An organization can only be successful if it has very good bedrock of policy, procedure and process.

> By the time CHI arrived here the senior management team had perhaps lost interest in this hospital. They were all looking for their next job, they all wanted glamorous national roles.

Learning and reflexive practice

An external report on the management of quality in the organization noted that some directorates and teams within Trust A had fostered a supportive environment for reporting clinical incidents and errors, but overall there had not generally been an open, learning environment in which staff felt confident about reporting problems. In the interviews many staff confirmed that a 'blame culture' existed under the previous regime which militated against reporting of mistakes,

clinical incidents and near misses. There was a strong feeling
that those admitting to mistakes would be scapegoated even
when the error was systemic in nature:

> It was very much a blame culture and it was always
> someone else's fault and the buck used to go down
> through the organization until there was a suitable
> place for it to stop, but it never went up.

> In the past you fill in the adverse events form and some-
> thing awful happened. You fill it in either nothing hap-
> pens or someone says – 'that was your fault, what did
> you do that for, that was a ridiculous thing to do.'

> There was definitely a feeling under the last administra-
> tion that if you made a mistake the trust would look
> after itself first.

A specific clinical incident was mentioned frequently in the
interviews and it was suggested that the managerial
response to this error sent a strong signal to staff that if they
owned up to errors or near misses they would be blamed
personally:

> There was a drug error to two patients in a row. It was a
> system error waiting to happen and was to do with
> drug labelling and packaging. And the individual clini-
> cians were sent on 'garden leave', pending investiga-
> tion. There was a very knee jerk response from the trust
> and someone had to be blamed. It sent a signal
> throughout the trust – Do Not Report Drug Errors that
> you might make or else you are gonna be treated in this
> way. The people at the senior management level now
> admit that wasn't handled well.

> The whole department were outraged at the way that
> [the clinical incident] had been dealt with and people
> said 'Well, you know I make 10,000 decisions a year
> and if I make a one per cent error rate then that is a hell
> of a lot of errors I am making. And if everytime I make
> one of those errors this happens then I'm not going to

report it.' So it was exactly counter to what we were being educated to do.

When confronted with information which showed that the trust was not performing well in a particular area, it was reported that the typical reaction from the core executive team was not to accept that there were problems and implement policies to remedy them, but rather to deny that any problem existed and to question the validity of the evidence. Thus, it would appear that the core executive team perpetuated and presided over an organizational culture that was far from conducive to learning and reflexive practice:

They [senior management team] usually dealt with criticism by saying it wasn't true . . . Or the people just didn't like [the chief executive] or us. It would be taken personally and there would be a view that the information that external people had was inaccurate. Which may well have been true actually because the information systems in the hospital are so bad.

There was a view here which was 'oh well we don't need to worry about that because we are [name of trust] darling and we're all rather fab and wonderful here so that doesn't involve us.' So there was an element of arrogance.

I can certainly remember going with [the previous chief executive] to Birmingham to teach new chief executives of PCTs the [name of trust] model and tell them how wonderful it is. It is very funny now and it's an embarrassment to think about it. The reality is that we portrayed this image that we were the best.

Many staff reported that some of the performance figures released by Trust A could not be trusted. Indeed at the time of the study the financial figures and waiting times data released by the trust were the subject of an investigation by external auditors. There were some concerns around accuracy of the data but some staff believed that performance data used for national ratings had been purposefully manipulated and misrepresented:

> As long as the figures were saying what the senior managers wanted them to say no one questioned how they were arrived at.

> One of the things trusts are measured on is 12 hour trolley wait. We reported no over 12 hour trolley waits when in fact we had them ... But if the information had been accurately put forward we would have been a no star trust.

> We had a finance director who could conceal things like it was going out of fashion.

> When I realized that the chief executive and director of finance were on the verge of moving on to another organization I whistle-blew on the organization. Went to the district auditors and said that the figures that were coming out at the recurring bottom line, we had significant financial problems which were being hidden. We were using non-recurring monies and we were robbing the next financial year to pay for the previous financial year.

External relationships

Trust A had faced a difficult and complex situation relating to relationships with key external stakeholders within the health economy. At the time of the study it related to several health authorities and a large number of primary care trusts and local authorities. There were some 'personality problems' between senior staff and external organizations. In particular there was a long history of antagonism between the trust and primary care services in the area which some staff believed may have affected continuity of care arrangements across the local health community which had served to increase re-admission rates to the trust.

Culture change policies initiated by the new chief executive

The purposeful management of the organization's culture was viewed as a crucial element of the new chief executive's strategy for improving the performance of the trust. To this end the incoming chief executive had instigated a review of decision making, accountability and communication.

The new chief executive was perceived by many to be more transactional and open in his approach to managing the organization. There was more of a focus on performance management issues and developing a supportive and learning culture across Trust A:

> Well [the new chief executive] is a very different style of person. [Chief executive] is very hands on. He is much more inclusive and open. He asks for feedback and listens to it from what I can see.

> There is a very striking difference between the new and old chief executive. The new chief executive has said on many occasions our culture for dealing with critical incidents will be judged by the way the next one is handled. There was definitely a feeling with the last administration that if you made a mistake the trust would look after itself first.

> A learning culture has to be open and transparent and the culture before was not. We now have open staff meetings and me sitting in front of the staff for an hour for them to fire questions at me is a good way of doing that.

> We now have 360% feedback for consultants where they get feedback from nurses and trainees. The implication in the past was that no nurse had anything to say that a doctor would find interesting.

There was a feeling amongst staff that external intervention (e.g. by the Modernisation Agency and the CHI review) had had a very positive effect on the organization and staff, not least because it had helped to 'cast a spotlight on' deficiencies within the trust which the previous senior management regime had chosen to ignore or 'sweep under the carpet'. The new chief executive viewed external checking and audit not only as a facilitator of public accountability but also as a tool to lever internal change.

Staff identified a range of potential problems around implementing cultural change programmes. First, there were difficulties in relation to finding resources and time to implement reforms when the organization was under extreme pressure to 'turn around' its performance. Second, many members of the old regime still occupied senior positions within the trust and there was a belief that these people were impeding constructive change within the organization. Finally, the wider NHS culture was believed to be at odds sometimes with the promotion of a 'no blame culture' within the organization. In particular the 'naming and shaming' of poorly performing trusts as part of the annual 'star' performance ratings was thought to be very unhelpful in this respect:

> The first problem is that virtually none of the clinical directors of [the previous chief executive's] regime have changed and that's something I said to [the new chief executive] he really needs to think about . . . so whatever happens he's going to have to change the people.

> I think it's an uphill struggle [implementing culture change] it's like swimming through treacle . . . it could take five years before cultures change. External factors have an influence as well, the culture throughout the NHS. We're part of an even bigger organization and the politicians have to accept a responsibility that there is a blame culture. Senior politicians want to blame doctors for what goes wrong.

Although the new chief executive had only been in post a short time there was a feeling by some that he had already had a positive impact on the culture of the organization:

the culture has changed immeasurably already [since the previous CE] . . . there's an openness now that we didn't have before. The cliques and the cabals are gradually being eviscerated.

There's been something like a two- or three-fold increase in the numbers of incidents reported. And that is partly down to the new forms – which are easy to use; partly down to education; and partly down to the fact that there is a genuine belief that they are supported. And we have had some red incidents that have been reported to the National Patient Safety Agency where individual members of staff have **not** been blamed.

Concluding remarks

Many of the problems at Trust A appear to stem from the leadership style of the previous chief executive and the apparent disconnection of the senior management team from the wider interest of the organization. In focusing on external opportunities, insufficient attention had been directed towards developing robust internal performance management processes and a 'climate of fear' had hung over the organization under which many staff were afraid to challenge senior management decisions or report adverse incidents and near misses. The new chief executive viewed culture change as a key element in the trust's strategy for improving performance and he was also viewed as cultivating a more inclusive and participatory approach to managing the trust. Although the new chief executive had been in post only a few months (and therefore possibly subject to a honeymoon effect) there was a general feeling that significant shifts in culture had already been achieved. Senior management was perceived as less cliquey and the blame culture appeared to be lifting, as evidenced by a large increase in reported clinical incidents.

TRUST B   MERGER MUDDLE

This trust which comprises a network of hospitals was formed less than five years prior to the study through the merger of two established trusts. It was assessed as 'low' performing (one or zero stars) in the performance ratings. There have recently been several key changes at a senior management level in the organization, including the appointment of a new chief executive. Key emergent themes from this case study include the problems that arise from the merger of health care organizations with very different management cultures; the dysfunctional consequences induced by the 'star' performance ratings; and the potential for bullying and harassment of staff to occur when senior managers are under pressure to turn around an under-performing organization. As the performance measures reported for the trust were the responsibility of the previous chief executive we first focus on the culture of the trust under this chief executive. We then explore the culture change strategies being implemented under the new chief executive.

Difficulties associated with the merger

Many of the staff interviewed reported that some of Trust B's difficulties were rooted in the merger. The two merged trusts (hereafter Trust Large and Trust Small) had very different organizational structures, management styles and established patterns of working. It appears that a residue of these differences survived the merger and served to stifle collaborative working across the two main hospital sites. It is interesting to note that staff appropriated the phrase '*us and them culture*' to describe the rift that was perceived to exist between the two former sites. Staff reported that there was considerable animosity between staff working on the two main sites, not least because of a perception by staff (working on the site which formerly comprised Trust Large) that resources had been diverted from their own services to cover the financial problems inherited from Trust Small:

Trust Large used to be an associated teaching hospital with no history of financial difficulties and an established reputation for good all round performance. It was suggested that staff in Trust Large felt resentful that they were having to 'bail out' Trust Small.

Trust Small are in a better financial situation now than they had ever been before the merger because there were huge financial problems which we had to bail out. And that is something people felt bitter about: 'I've worked hard – I've developed my service' and then people on the other side were saying 'oh I need money – I haven't got money to do this' . . . So there was a feeling of expecting us to bail them out and why should we – that was very difficult. It was hard for them and it was hard for Trust Small as well. So I'm sounding like a 'them and us' culture, and it *is* very easy to slip into that. You talk about them, and you talk about us.

There was a real buzz to the place [Trust Large], then we merged and there was a kind of 'them and us' [a prevailing view that] they are going to pull us down. We're in the black but they are in the red. We're going to have to pick up their losses.

There was clearly a tension between the Trusts . . . the cultures are very different and because we're pussyfooting around each other it becomes very difficult to put those cultures together.

Staff reported considerable practical and political problems around setting and delivering an effective organization-wide performance management agenda. Not just animosity between senior managers across the two main hospital sites, but in addition the patient administration systems on the two sites were not 'communicating with each other', and staff grading and remuneration packages differed across the trust, prompting further tensions.

Some of the problems in creating a cohesive approach to the organization's performance management arose from inherited differences in approaches to corporate and clinical governance across the two main hospital sites. Trust Large had an established clinical directorate structure in which responsibility and decision making was devolved to professional teams. In contrast, Trust Small was viewed as more of a 'centralist' organization with relatively few devolved freedoms and flexibilities. Trust Small was perceived by some as being slower to modernize, redesign its traditional modes of working and sign up fully to implementing the new corporate agenda:

> We [Trust Large] had a completely different management structure from Trust Small. Ours is very devolved: take responsibility; push it down as low as you can. Trust Small is very centrally managed. So when they merged it was a huge culture shock for Trust Small.

> The Trust Small consultant body are organized more as group of clinicians. They communicate well with each other – they have a slightly more united front . . . [In this hospital] I would say there is not as good communication between consultants. At the Trust Small end they never did have a devolved structure, and it was only after being merged that development took place. At Trust Small the culture was very much a centralist one, everything happened from the chief executive's office. If you wanted something you went to talk to him about it. In a sense it was a benign dictatorship.

> At the other end of the hospital [Trust Small] the problem is not that they are not prepared to take risks – in fact they are quite risk takers – but they've become very entrenched in refusing to change, because they see all change as threatening to them.

Leadership styles and management orientation

The previous chief executive at Trust B was considered a good theoretician but lacking the requisite transactional skills and strategic vision to set up and run an effective trust-wide performance management system. He was also said to have failed to 'win the hearts and minds' of staff or harness the full potential of the workforce to improve the organization's performance.

> [The previous chief executive's] leadership was fundamentally different from [the current chief executive's]. [The previous chief executive] was a very intelligent theorist and that in the end was part of the problem – the theory just grounded. He just couldn't *do* something.

> There was no direction, no leadership and, I think, panic – because it was all going wrong, and no one knew how to fix it.

> Dominant cultural trait of the trust? 'Can't do' – that's my first impression [new chief executive speaking]. Very few people came with ideas about good solutions to problems.

Under the previous regime performance management was considered to be the main responsibility of individual directorates and there appeared to be a very relaxed approach to holding clinical directors accountable for their performance. As mentioned above, an external report on the management of the organization had used the term 'us and them culture' to describe the disconnection that apparently existed between the senior management team and the rest of the organization. Our study lends support to this view. Some interviewees reported that the senior management team had become remote and inaccessible, seen as more interested in pursuing their personal agendas than interacting with staff lower down the hierarchy:

> The trust's view on performance management was what I'd call collective management, which was

focused on some areas of performance – but in a very two dimensional way. So there were performance meetings which looked at figures but didn't in my view really relate [these] to what has to happen in the service to make the figures happen.

There wasn't a planning culture . . . there were encouraged to be self-running directorates who competed with each other. But now I want them [new chief executive speaking] to co-operate with each other . . . to be a whole system.

We used to have a review meeting where we met with the executive team about every six weeks. They were relaxed meetings . . . it was an opportunity to discuss how we are doing. What we have now [under the new chief executive] is an operational review meeting. 'These are the things we want you to report on.' It's pages of score charts which go into every detail.

The senior management were invisible to the rest of the organization. Before I came [the new chief executive speaking] the culture was one of invisibility. No one ever walked around the trust.

Our study identified a perception that the tier of middle management at the organization had been under-developed and senior managers frequently neglected to draw on the experience and expertise of middle managers when planning and implementing trust policy.

When I arrived here I found basically a group of general managers who . . . were not very well developed . . . there was really a bunch of disenfranchised, disempowered general managers who were working like low level business managers.

I think we have a dearth of talent here which is historical at a middle management level . . . So with all the best will in the world I would say I've got some

managers who are doing very well – but none are out-
standing in any sense.

Accountability and use of information

Accountability within Trust B was far from clear and
transparent, particularly in terms of quality assurance and
clinical governance arrangements. Although, the medical
director had taken the lead in implementing the trust's clinical governance agenda he did not have the benefit of a
dedicated support team to back up his efforts. An external
report on the organization had noted that although the
clinical governance board met regularly, and produced
minutes and reports, these did not appear to have been
disseminated to staff expected to implement policy.
Although the trust did operate an appraisal system for staff,
it was perceived by many staff to be more punitive than
developmental.

> We did have tight control, and we would be given very
> clear indicators as to how we were doing financially.

> They [the senior management team] lost touch with
> each other. They didn't have management team meet-
> ings, they had update meetings – but didn't discuss
> what they could do as a team. They just told each other
> what they were doing, and used to meet for an hour
> once a week.

> Clinical quality [information systems] we are not happy
> with at all, and we are starting to do some work on
> that. They seem to be happy with the financial informa-
> tion. But when it comes down to clinical quality infor-
> mation, there's very little of that.

> The IT information systems are [still] a bit creaky . . .
> You can run the same report on consecutive days and it
> comes up with different figures, it is very bizarre.

> There have always been gaps in terms of who is respon-
> sible for what.

Learning and reflexive practice

Although Trust B publicly espoused a 'no blame' policy it was reported that the culture was such that staff did not feel confident in openly reporting clinical errors and untoward incidents for fear of recrimination. There was a widespread belief that this 'blame culture' resulted in a serious under-reporting of clinical incidents in the organization and therefore deterred learning and reflexive practice.

> Another part of the culture about 'can't do' was 'don't tell'. That was a real problem here. People never reported anything. A nurse would never think about reporting a doctor or even just raising concerns in a team meeting.

> I found it a bit disappointing that we're supposed to be a learning organization. So if someone makes a mistake you should be able to say 'well, I've made a mistake – how can we retrieve this?' – but [instead] it's the philosophy 'oh, get it wrong and you're out!'

> It is very difficult, especially where the targets are not directly related to patient benefit . . . we all care about patient benefit but us having to concentrate on this target doesn't actually do it. The worst people in the world for cultivating a blame culture are CHI and the centre. 'You are failing your targets so we'll sack you' . . . that doesn't actually tie in with what they are preaching for the rest of us to do.

> Appraisal wasn't done particularly well in the directorates, so people would see it as quite threatening rather than [as] rewarding and recognizing good work.

External relationships

An external report on Trust B noted that there was a lack of openness about the functions of partnerships with external organizations and patients, and that this had impacted on effective communications with partner organizations. It also reported that local community health councils felt that their views were not actively sought and there was little evidence that progress had been made in involving the public in consultation about services. However it did point out that there were good relationships with social care organizations and community hospitals. One positive outcome of the external review (not withstanding the major reservations above) was a feeling that it had helped to open up better lines of communication with a range of organizations in the local health economy:

> One of the positive aspects of the [external] report was that we knew it was coming, and just prior to its public release we had a stakeholder meeting . . . [where] we had representation of the health authorities, the PCGs, the Community Health Council . . . That engagement sowed the seeds for a lot of communication . . . and they are continuing to be engaged in various ways.

Dysfunctional consequences

There was a strong feeling amongst staff at Trust B that the external review and the poor star rating assessment had tarnished the trust's reputation and that this had a deleterious impact on staff morale. The external review was reported to have had the knock-on effect of damaging relationships with patients and within the wider health economy. It appears that a vitriolic media campaign waged against the trust had exacerbated the situation and fired local hostility towards staff. Some staff believed the trust had contributed to its plight by not preparing sufficiently for the review and there was a feeling that it would have achieved a more favourable report (and thus a higher star rating) if it had focused on highlighting the more successful services at the trust. Several staff commented that the external review document did not portray a balanced view of the trust. For example it was thought that undue weight had been given to isolated comments at public meetings (e.g. concerning dirty wards), or the fact that some visits by external reviewers to individual departments had been pre-scheduled, thus allowing them to fare relatively well in the assessment as they had been able to 'window-dress' in preparation:

> This organization was pretty naïve at the time [of the review] because we were one of the first few organizations to be done. I think they didn't know what to expect, and didn't know how to sell themselves or sell the positive things.

> [The public perception was] 'You go to [name of trust] and you die!' We had people on the wards demanding the self-discharge forms and getting crushed in the rush to leave . . . It was just awful – nurses demanding changing rooms because they didn't want to go outside the trust [in uniform] because they were being accosted in the streets . . . and in the shops people were saying 'God you don't work for that place do you? How many have you killed today?'

> What we all recognize is that reputations can take a very long time to build up but can be dashed in an instant.

> It was devastating [the low star rating]. It was the worst thing that could have happened. The [external] report was bad enough. It was unfair – what drags people down is the unfairness of it . . . Even they were surprised, and didn't expect the media reaction. And there have been far worse reports written since and before which didn't get that much media coverage . . . We knew our jobs were on the line there. But the stars was the last straw and hit right down to the workforce – whereas bad reports usually hit senior management upwards.

Culture change policies initiated under the new chief executive

The new chief executive at Trust B was viewed as having a more practical 'hands on' approach to managing the trust than his predecessor. Indeed, he was considered by many to possess the transactional skills required to turn around under-performance in the trust. A key difference is that more senior management time and energy was devoted to ensuring that the trust was meeting external performance targets. The new approach depended on a system of subsidiary where upward accountability to the centre for performance was strengthened but more freedom and autonomy was devolved to 'high' performing service directorates. Efforts were also being made to eradicate the 'us and them' culture that was said to have existed between senior managers and the wider organization. There was a recognition by senior managers that a major culture change initiative was required to overcome the entrenched differences between the two main trust sites and a package of measures were being introduced to improve communication and facilitate joint working across the whole organization. New emphasis was also placed on developing an empowered tier of middle management and on nurturing a team-based approach to securing performance improvements.

> The whole essence is organizational culture [chief executive speaking]. You can bring things together on a service basis but if people don't want to change and see a bigger organization as a whole rather than two separate halves then it is difficult. That is the real challenge that I face.

> In this directorate we run speciality meetings which are cross-site. We alternate consultant meetings between sites and there is plenty of encouragement for people to work together. When we are satisfied that people are working well together then we merge their budgets, but it is a minority at the moment.

> There's been a very big change in the way that beds are managed – a very much tightening up in procedures which is why we've done very well on the trolley waits . . . All this started to happen with the appointment of the new chief executive.

Now it is completely target driven . . . before we had more autonomy. I was a general manager, and how I managed the programme was really up to me . . . perhaps we were a little too casual in some respects. But now it's run in completely the opposite way.

A lot of people still say – despite the fact that there is, I think there is, better communication than there was between senior management and the rest of the trust – a lot of people still think senior management is remote . . . It's being worked on very hard and the executive directors do try and get out and talk to people a lot more than ever happened before but it's a slow process.

And what I've tried to do [new chief executive speaking] is bring quite a strong degree of central control in – but with appropriate delegated authority. So I encourage people to work within a framework.

A lot of people still think senior management is remote. I do think it's getting better and all the things I've said about [the new chief executive's] open attitude is much appreciated but I think there's still a 'them and us culture'.

But people have to deliver. Fairness doesn't come into it [chief executive speaking]. That's not meant to be a macho response . . . there is quite a lot of support around . . . but I haven't found a way of dealing with the resisters apart from saying this is what we want and this is what you'll deliver.

It has been approached in a different way from the way we did it three years ago [during the merger]. There's been a great deal more clinician and stakeholder involvement.

We've changed the senior managers' objective setting process. Instead of having team-set objectives – which was in some ways good because they encourage team work, but actually they also encourage people to sit out and let other people do it and then not to bother – so we are setting much more personal objectives.

On a more negative note there was a feeling among some staff that the emphasis on delivering measurable improvements in performance had contributed to a culture of 'bullying' staff. It was suggested that as senior staff were under increasing pressures to hit national performance targets, they were sometimes resorting to threats and intimidation to achieve the desired improvements. The focus on meeting external performance targets was reported to have distorted clinical priorities because of the need to focus on areas of measured performance to the detriment of other important but unmeasured areas of clinical activity. It was suggested that this was contributing to a growing tension between the consultant body and senior managers, and between senior managers and middle managers:

I was quite shocked by the senior managers and the terminology they use ... if we didn't achieve our targets 'heads would roll and desks would be cleared' – and it wasn't said jokingly, it was said quite seriously.

It's acute pressure that's never been there before to achieve the targets. And I think it's a sort of panic reaction – people start shouting and screaming at everyone else 'Do it! Do it! Do it!' Well we can't.

It's just ironic that in the [external] report they talked about the bullying culture within the trust, which no one recognized ... It just wasn't that type of culture at all ... So people say 'well, we didn't have one – so bring one in!' You know, screaming and shouting – I've never had it in all my years of working ... This is what is so ironic: we talk about it has to be 'no blame', and the person that is saying there has to be a 'no blame culture' can then turn around and say 'if you get it wrong it's curtains for you' ... that's the message coming down from higher up. It's a sham.

The culture's changed. It's not so much about if we achieve all these stars we can become a foundation hospital – which is what I'd like to hear – it's [so-and-

so's] job is on the line or . . . if you don't do this it will
be 'curtains for you' . . . It's all very different to the
culture we are used to, which has come as a very rude
awakening.

It is completely target driven now, and what is difficult
is that the targets are so conflicting . . . the fact that we
can't have patients waiting in A&E and therefore we
have to protect more beds in case people come in
through A&E . . . affects the ability for us to bring our
[own elective] patients in . . . Consultants are saying
[that] if this happen again they'll go and discharge your
patient and bring in my patient. And we've been told
that, and as hard as this is, that we won't have the
Department or Region on our back.

More emphasis was now being placed on the collection
and use of timely, accurate and valid data to support clinical
governance. Specific initiatives were also being developed
to ensure trust-wide compatibility of IT procurements and
enhance the IT skills of staff where appropriate. The trust was
also developing a 'balanced scorecard' approach to monitoring clinical processes and outcomes and it was believed that
this would inform the development of benchmarking of the
trust's services over time and assist comparisons with similar
trusts. Most of these initiatives are, however, in their early
days:

We are just about to introduce a balanced scorecard, a
monthly assessment of performance. And that makes
it clear who is responsible for performance. There is a
lot of clarity . . . [before] it was a monthly meeting
with the trust exec to see how you were getting on.
There was no fixed agenda. It is much more structured
now.

We're using a balanced scorecard . . . [and] we are trying to develop some of the clinical performance issues
as well. There's work we are doing with the directorates
to ensure that meeting performance gets away from
the old fashioned [focus on] activity and money.

We've just had [some detailed] patient data, and we've looked at the top eight problem areas, so we'll be doing something specific around them. We've also just purchased a better system for looking at complaints in different groups . . . We've also done focus groups.

A number of potential barriers to implementing change in the organization were identified. These included the difficulties in trying to make changes without removing key staff from their current positions and the fact that change required a level of risk that some staff were reluctant to take:

It is very difficult to change cultures without changing personalities. And I think the three new directors from outside the trust and myself . . . do bring a very different 'can do' culture into the trust.

We're meeting resistance but not because people don't like the things we can do. I think it is that they just don't yet feel equipped to be able to take that sort of risk.

Concluding remarks

Many of Trust B's performance difficulties appear to stem from the merger of two trusts with very different established traditions of working. These differences impeded collaborative working and served to engender an adversarial 'us and them' culture within the organization. Poor external assessments and adverse media coverage had also served to erode staff morale. The new chief executive was attempting to improve communication across the organization and senior management were placing new emphasis on delivering the external performance management agenda. However, we heard reports that this new approach had created a 'culture of bullying' with some managers using threats and intimidation to effect the desired improvements. Therefore, this case study highlights the importance of attending to cultural as well as structural issues in health service re-organization; and the need to monitor carefully the policies, tactics and incentives used by managers (and external agencies) to 'turnaround' performance in 'low' performing trusts.

TRUST C   GET A GRIP

Trust C is a modern district general hospital providing services across a broad range of medical and surgical specialties. It was classified as low performing (awarded zero or one star) in the NHS performance ratings. There have been several recent changes to the executive and non-executive members of the trust board. As the performance measures reported for the Trust were the responsibility of the previous chief executive we first focus on the culture of the trust under this chief executive. We then explore the culture change strategies being implemented under the new chief executive.

Leadership style and management orientation

The previous senior management team at Trust C was described as a collection of very committed and personable individuals. However the senior management team appears to have adopted a very relaxed approach to managing the organization and many believed that they lacked the transactional skills required to establish robust internal performance management systems. The senior management teams were believed to function poorly as a team and some thought that individual members were more focused on pursuing their own 'empire building' and 'pet projects' than on concentrating on the wider interests of the organization:

> When I first started [current chief executive speaking] it was a management that was entirely focused on its financial efforts. Not operating as a team. There were certain people pursuing their own agendas and there wasn't a common agenda for the trust. I'm afraid there's going to have to be some casualties along the way but I came to the conclusion that some people will never change their ways.

> It was very laid back [the organization]. It was very friendly but it never hit the hard deliverables. The

recover plan was put in place by that management team but had to be carried through by the current team.

[Under the previous regime] people were less stressed, people were happy, there were less restriction.

The comment I would make about the previous regime was that it thought 'it would be alright on the day' and no one would make hard decisions. You used to come out of meetings and say 'for God's sake someone please do something'. He was a delightful chap, we all liked him immensely but you just felt there was no cutting edge there. When the new regime came in there were some tough decisions made and some people didn't like it but things moved.

The previous management were very friendly but didn't get anywhere. Trying to please everybody. When asked for something he [the chief executive] would say 'yes, no problem' but didn't get anywhere. Things didn't move as fast as they do now.

When I came here one of my first tasks as [job title] was to find out what other people's perceptions of the job were . . . I went to regions and said 'well what's your perception of the trust?' And the perception was that it's a bit of a sleepy organization and hasn't stirred itself. So there were a few comments like 'that trust's has always been thinking about this but has never actually done it'.

Prior to [the current chief executive] the senior management team operated in isolation. Their directorates were sufficiently large and powerful that whatever the other senior manager said they didn't have to play ball.

It was reported that senior management attention had focused primarily on meeting external financial and waiting list targets and that this had directed energy and resources

away from developing effective clinical governance arrangements for the trust. These comments support an external
report on the organization which stated that although the
board had many good ideas around clinical governance
these had not been effectively embedded within the organization. In particular clinical governance activities were not
part of an integrated programme of quality assurance and
improvement and in some areas were perceived as being
peripheral to core operational activity:

> They have been focused on their financial problems but
> in doing that I think they've actually neglected the
> vision of where they wanted to be.

> In the past the performance of the hospital, under
> whatever parameters you measure, I mean financial per-
> formance, waiting lists, waiting targets – all these were
> very much a function of the financial mess we were in.
> And that's where the focus was not clinical areas.

There was a general feeling that the middle tier of management had been under-developed over many years and that
this had hampered the organization's ability to develop and
deliver robust systems of performance management. In particular it was felt that there should have been greater middle
management input to support the clinical directorates.

> This trust is extremely lean on management and I think
> we suffered for it [clinician speaking]. I think we are
> now in a situation of trying to turn that around.

> Our management review has identified that at the level
> of clinical directorates we are under-strength. They
> actually produce the day-to-day business.

> They didn't have the support they needed from man-
> agers who could have told them a thing or two and
> not got the organization into the mess it found itself
> in . . . this is something which needs attention now if
> we are not to be condemned to repeating these same
> mistakes.

Staff talked of a tension existing between executive and non-executive members on the trust board. There was a feeling (by executives) that non-executives exerted an undue influence over day-to-day operational matters at the hospital and some believed that there was an agenda by the non-executives on the board to replace executives currently in post:

> One of the biggest mistakes we make in this organization, and I know the chairman will totally disagree with me, is that we put non-execs as chairmen of sub-committees in the trust board. So all decisions have to go through them.

> The execs don't trust the non-execs at all – there is great suspicion. There's been a feeling in the past that the non-execs have been out to undermine the execs and that there is a hidden agenda and they want certain of them out – That the non-execs want to run the organization and don't know their place.

Accountability and use of information

Information systems, particularly those useful to supporting the clinical governance agenda had been under-developed in Trust C. There was a feeling by some that the lack of accurate and timely information was the root cause of many of the trust's problems. An external report on the organization noted that although the trust board received information on such matters as waiting times and complaints, the quality of clinical data was poor. Clinical staff reported a lack of routinely produced information, which would help them to monitor their patient outcomes and to enable them to measure their performance. A number of examples were identified where clinicians had developed their own databases to supplement the inadequacies of the information system.

Specific roles and responsibilities of senior staff were not always clear and in some areas overlapped and in others there were serious gaps. This situation was felt by some to have undermined the development of a co-ordinated approach to performance management across the trust. An external report on the organization noted, however, that at a corporate and clinical team level staff interviewed demonstrated a clear understanding of their roles and this was supported by job descriptions:

> When I arrived here there was not a systematic approach across the organization to recording clinical incidents.

> Our information system is poor and that is the root cause of a lot of our problems.

> IT is a major problem and we are trying to address it. There's been a history that IT was shelved. When we were short of money that is the thing that was missed. Computer technology is now one of our priorities but it's taking a hell of a long time to get it sorted out.

> Money was taken out of developing information systems for monitoring activity . . . it never appeared as a priority for them [the senior management team] . . . If I had had my way we would have invested more heavily in this rather than pursue some of the more hare-brained schemes we were expected to go along with.

> We made mistakes that got us a one star that we should have handled. We had the information at our fingertips. We didn't action and think it through.

Human resources policies

Trust C had a history of difficulties in recruiting staff in some clinical areas and there were serious shortfalls in the number of nursing staff employed. It was felt that this impacted deleteriously on the quality of patient care. An external report noted a concern over the retention and sickness levels at the trust. The report contained accounts of staff citing stress at work and lowering of job satisfaction combined with an increase in workload as significant factors in the high level of sickness at the trust. Staff morale was reported to be variable across the organization with low morale demonstrated in areas where high workload and staff shortfalls were reported. And there were a number of areas where staff felt unsupported and were unconvinced of the priority attached to this at board level, expressing the view that staff morale was secondary to the achievement of targets:

> Basically, we are appointing whoever we can get. And in many specialities if we can get anybody who is vaguely going to do the job, we grab them.

> We don't really think about managing the human resources angle too much. If they apply and we have a vacancy then more often than not they get the job with no questions asked.

> A lot of the nurses in particular are dissatisfied with the amount of work and cover they have to put in . . . it's getting a little better now but we have been under-resourced in this area and patients have not always been getting as good a care environment as they could and deserve.

Culture change policies implemented by the new chief executive

The new chief executive at Trust C was described as a transactional leader with a clear focus on delivering on key performance targets and modernizing the organization around the needs of patients. There was a shift towards making individual directorates more accountable for their performance and devolving power down to directorate level to enable staff to be more creative in how they design services around the needs of patients. There was also a strong feeling by some staff that the chairman was a key driving influence behind the new performance management agenda and some believed that he might be the 'power behind the throne' and forcing through a radical agenda of change management:

The strategy that we've developed is very much a top down strategy.

I think the culture of the management team is very positive.

We are undertaking a management review because we need to change our focus and structure to be able to adapt more quickly to the NHS plan and the national agenda.

You have to be driven by targets and if you want to go after something, you cannot let it drift. You've got to be focused and get it.

Change makes people feel uncomfortable. People generally like to be left to themselves. And as an organization I think we need people to lift them out of those comfort zones.

[Referring to the current chief executive] Very, very good at interpersonal skills, very approachable, very relaxed. He turned around a very difficult organization. He changed the structure and how it operated. Made the directorates more accountable. Gave them far more devolved power and made them accept the responsibility that went along with that.

Some people feel that the new management is a bit pushy . . . but if you want to make hard decisions you need to be unpopular at times.

He is not a rubber stamper [chairman] let's put it that way. He is actively involved, he listens and is very sharp. Most of the people in the Trust respect the chairman, they do.

[In five years' time] the senior management team will have changed quite dramatically. We will see a lot of change. I think the chairman will have quite a profound effect on the organization and [the chief executive] as well. And I would like to feel in five years' time that we will have a much more open culture where staff feel safe to report problems and feel they are involved in the organization.

We are short on management capacity and the exec team do too much operational work. In terms of performance management we've done too much trying to deliver the targets on the ground. I've done deals with consultants. I shouldn't be doing deals with consultants. I've been chivvying them along. I shouldn't be doing that. There's a huge development need in the middle tier and it needs restructuring and resourcing better.

However some people held reservations about the leadership style of the new chief executive and other members of the senior management team. Some senior clinicians were concerned that the focus on meeting the performance management agenda was distorting clinical priorities and others, whilst acknowledging the positive contribution of the chief executive, did not believe that he possessed the 'ruthlessness' required to overcome the various institutional and professional barriers that prevented change in the organization. There also appeared to still be some tension between the members of the senior management team and this appeared to be fuelled, in part, by a perception that some would be replaced in the near future:

There is definitely too much attention focused on that [meeting national targets] and that is where clinical priorities go out of the window.

[The current chief executive] has been very successful in moving this organization forward and there has been a lot of investment in the organization and the whole waiting list issue has been addressed. But it's almost as if there is something within his personality that is not as good. I've seen it before, perhaps someone who's been an arch bastard in the past and he's had a sort of road to Damascus experience and is perhaps scared to go back to that arch bastard situation. I think he just needs to take a much firmer line in some situations.

The rest of the senior management team is quite dysfunctional and there have been lots of problems. They are a bunch of prima donnas that's the best way to describe them. They are scoring points off each other and back-stabbing and it is a very difficult environment to work in.

We are trying to empower directorates. They haven't had the wherewithal to do what they needed to do.

Improving the provision and use of computerized information within the organization is a key element in the Trust's agenda for addressing the information difficulties of the trust. A special subcommittee of the Trust board had been established to implement the policy, which is chaired by the trust's chairman and includes representation from each directorate. At the time of the study all clinical staff had access to the Internet via either a dedicated personal computer or a shared PC. In addition an Internet café for staff use was to be set up in the near future.

Policies were being put in place to attempt to embed more of an open 'no blame' culture within the organization. The director of nursing had lead responsibility for developing training for staff in this area and increasing the understanding and compliance of medical staff in reporting incidents. One of the policies involved the induction process for junior staff to be improved. Others included the appointment of a dedicated clinical risk manager and the development of computer software to capture and disseminate rapidly emerging trends in clinical incident reporting throughout the Trust. Staff reported that, although the trust had made significant strides in nurturing a no blame culture, there was still someway to go before many staff felt safe to report adverse incidents and near misses:

The culture of this hospital is that we try to be open, we try to be honest, we try to keep people informed.

We're not there yet. We have not got a no blame culture yet through the organization. There are people in this organization, I am sure, who have concerns about their work that they cannot say anything or do anything about.

We still haven't got used to clinical incidence reporting at this trust.

We are now trying to feed back to people the outcome of incidents that are reported. That is something we'd forgotten to do in the past.

There exist and persist problems around reporting adverse events because some of the fundamental problems in the systems and people in post ... meaning how people talk and react to each other in certain situations here ... Sometimes it's like banging your head against a brick wall asking staff to report things for us to learn and improve on ... There's a legacy from another era which means they won't do it no matter how much we tell them to.

A focus of management attention was on implementing and developing of Trust C's new appraisal process. This was viewed as a key mechanism for developing more of a corporate culture amongst health professionals, especially junior doctors and consultants. The formal appraisal of all consultants had been completed in the previous year and departmental training plans had been revised to demonstrate a stronger link between departmental and directorate objectives, as well as the staff's training and development needs that are identified through the appraisal process. To complete the training cycle a status report is used as a tool to highlight key training activity undertaken within each directorate and to evaluate its effectiveness and impact on service delivery. A training needs analysis had also recently been undertaken with clinical directors to identify their development needs in relation to management skills needed to undertake the managerial aspects of their role. There was, however, some concerns over the continuation of a 'bullying culture' at the trust and some staff believed that this was being exacerbated by the pressures placed on staff to deliver on the national targets:

> A new system of staff appraisal which is important because that starts to change the culture of getting people to talk about each other and getting staff's objectives lined up with the organization's objectives.

> People have said that they've been bullied and hassled in the past and I think there still is a culture of that in the organization and it needs to be dealt with.

> There is more pressure to perform well on performance indicators . . . it is not as nice a place to work in as everyone is looking over their backs to see if they are for the chop or not.

External relationships

Trust C had a history of poor relationships with other local organizations. This was due in part to 'personality differences' between senior managers in partner organizations. However it was reported that over the previous year, senior managers had sought to improve relationships with other organizations and to contribute more positively towards 'actively managing' the local health economy:

> I think we increasingly need to understand how their organizations function [other organizations in the local health community]. For example the local authority – I've never had a clue how they function. I've never been interested. I've got enough on trying to understand this one without trying to understand someone else's. But we are increasingly looking to improve our relationships.

> We were not seen as a high profile player . . . We now

have meetings with PCTs social services. People are seeing us now as a bigger player purely for raising that
profile.

Concluding comments

This case study highlights the role strong transactional management has in setting up robust internal performance management systems. The previous management at Trust C had
failed to invest in good information systems or to develop a
cadre of middle management capable of driving and delivering change on the ground. The internal rivalries between
members of the senior management team and non-
executives, and between different clinical directorates, also
appears to have had a negative impact on the functioning
and performance of the organization. The new chief executive was seeking to address this situation through a better
balance between transactional and transformational
approaches to managing the organization.

TRUST D   IN WITH THE IN CROWD

The Trust is a large acute teaching hospital providing a range
of specialist and teaching services. It was classified as a low
performing Trust (awarded a zero or one star) in the performance ratings. There have been several changes in key
senior staff at the trust over recent years, including a new
chief executive, chairman, director of nursing and finance
director. As the performance measures reported for the trust
were the responsibility of the previous chief executive we
first focus on the culture of the trust under that chief executive. We then explore the culture change strategies being
implemented under the new chief executive.

The previous management regime (although there had
been many changes in key staff and several chief executives
over the previous ten years) was described as being a type of
clique or cabal, headed by a charismatic chief executive in

which a few favoured members of a close knit inner circle made all the key decisions. The inner circle was viewed as being very disconnected and remote from the wider organization. This, it was suggested, was one of the root causes of the trust's problems as corporate policy was made without sufficient consultation and the support and advice of middle management. Many of the senior management team were also regarded as preoccupied with their own career and advancement rather than on the key issues facing the Trust. Rewards (both to individuals and to areas of speciality) were said to be largely based on patronage (i.e. closeness and loyalty to the inner circle) rather than based on transparent and objective measures of performance:

> The leadership was very different from now. There were many clinical directorates which encouraged a parochial approach by the then business managers and the clinical directors to 'look after their own patch'. The place was very much run by the chief executive who was advised by a very small group.

> Some clinical directors and directorates were favoured more than others. I think the 'in' groups were the specialities where investments were made . . . I certainly experienced less investment in my area as a result of my face not fitting.

> A lot of the senior managers in the old guard – board members – were looking for higher, better posts, rather than focusing on the here-and-now of the trust's difficulties.

> The [management] style was to divide and rule and he did it quite cleverly. Instead of having four clinical directorates he had thirteen . . . and you could be sure that [the number of clinical directorates] couldn't make any decisions . . . there were favourites and I think that is the origins of some of the trust's problems now.

It was reported that the senior management team some-times resorted to threats, intimidation and bullying to push forward their policies:

A lot of organizations I've gone to welcomed with open arms the [external assessments] visit because the senior management teams were very dysfunctional, who did have cliques, who did bully, who had all these prob-lems with the culture.

There wasn't so much bullying as 'if you don't do this then I can assure you that something much worse will happen'. That was the standard scenario, the set piece.

If you were not in with them then there was always this feeling that you would be out on your ear if you didn't do what they asked . . . I suppose it was a low level type of threatening culture which kept people in place without obviously doing so.

It appears that the main consultant body, apart from a few favoured senior clinicians in the inner circle, were largely excluded from participating in corporate decision making and strategy development. This led to problems over the planning of clinical services and served to alienate senior clinicians:

In the [previous senior management team] era there was certainly an alienation of the consultant staff from key decisions. There was a belief that they sat in this little cabal making the decisions. It was fine if you were one of the favourites.

One of the things that's been said about us is that we always take on developments without ensuring that the hospital has income for it and that was one of the reasons why it became financially unstable.

We had an extremely unwieldy executive board, with many clinical directorates it depended who was in favour. By some backdoor phenomenon you would

suddenly discover that there was a new vascular surgeon or a respiratory physician etc. There was no
formal input into strategy but you would suddenly
discover there was more work, more demand which
you hadn't be consulted about.

I think decisions were made for others. I think decisions
were made in an autocratic, non-inclusive way and
people had to succumb to these decisions.

We were forced to dance to their tune [senior management team] and were not considered.

Given the history of financial problems at the trust it was
reported that the key focus of the senior management team
was on seeking to meet the trust's financial recovery plan.
This focus on financial issues meant that clinical governance
arrangements were generally under-developed and under-
resourced:

In the previous senior management team, I was the
most junior member. I was appointed shortly before
people started leaving, which meant I was thrown in
at the deep end. There was a preoccupation with bal-
ancing the books. The main driver was financial rather
than keeping a check on what was happening on the
clinical side of things and how to improve patient
quality.

The Trust had a bad financial problem. The area the
board focused on was trying to balance the book year-
on-year, cost improvement programmes at 3 percent
year-on-year. And 'salami slicing' services because the
board held the view that if they were in financial balance that would secure development opportunities
and secure the future of the trust.

Accountability and use of information

Accountability in Trust D had been opaque and there was confusion over which senior staff were responsible for specific

areas of performance. This situation was exacerbated by the fact that the organization was structured across many clinical directorates, which made planning and co-ordination difficult. The focus on financial performance identified above diverted attention and resources away from developing robust systems of clinical governance across the trust. This made it very difficult for the senior management team to monitor both financial and clinical performance. Indeed, an external report on the organization noted that it was unclear how information relating to clinical governance was reviewed, evaluated and acted upon in the organization. The report also recognized that the status of information systems and technology infrastructure at the trust was seriously under-developed:

> There has been a serious under-investment in the financial and clinical IT systems in this trust. Because of the financial crisis the infrastructure and IT suffered. And I think there is now more recognition that we need to pump more money into that.

Learning and reflexive practice

It was reported that the old regime in Trust D had not nurtured a culture that was conducive to open reporting and learning from clinical errors and adverse incidents. Those found to have erred were said to be blamed or scapegoated and this sent a strong signal to staff not to report clinical incidents or own up to errors:

> On the nursing side there was a very disciplinarian approach to clinical incidents. Nurses were heavily disciplined and fired when things went wrong and that is something we are trying to get away from.

> It used to be the case that when something went wrong in the past it was hidden. I don't think many people were punished as much as kept very quiet. I think it is now very much more open but it has been a very difficult job.

A manager [senior nurse] flagged up a data type problem around clinical governance in the directorate. Well the manager was sacked or moved on depending on your view. The lessons are still being learnt. But I think what staff throughout the ranks took was here is someone who is doing a decent job or somebody who is quite good at their job and who flagged up an issue but was a scapegoat.

Current culture policies initiated by the new chief executive

The new chief executive was reported to be implementing wide ranging reforms which were believed to be gradually changing the culture of Trust D. He was described as a more participatory style of leader with a clear agenda to devolve power and responsibility down the organization. However, the chief executive was aware that a dose of transactional style leadership was required to establish robust systems and procedures to support performance management. The clinical directorates had been reduced to four to facilitate better co-ordination and team working across specialties. These clinical directorates were supported by several cross-cutting service directorates. However, an external report on the organization noted that there was still work to be done in bringing clinical teams and directorates together and seeing themselves jointly as part of a corporate structure. It also observed that there was a sense that directorates had created their own infrastructures and ways of working and operated to some degree almost independently of the wider organization:

I think anyone coming in to try and transform the place [the trust] – Well people just couldn't have coped with it. There was a sense of turmoil, and what was needed was stability. A bit of process, a bit of good old fashioned bureaucracy to build a sense of order in the way things were done. So I've been very keen to promote this leadership style [current chief executive speaking] and I try and promote involvement in, and ownership of, decisions.

It is moving more towards transformational stuff in that now we are becoming more explicitly value driven and we are saying – 'right we have some of the building blocks in place – what sort of organization do we want to be?' Having said that though there is still a significant infrastructure back-filling job.

We now have a new post of director of performance and modernization, who works closely with the chief executive.

I don't think it is a rigid type of leadership. I think it is a leadership which really believes in valuing people. There is a lot of effort now put into involving all staff at different levels in the running of the organization . . . it hasn't worked in all areas yet but hopefully it will soon.

There has been a big culture change within finance. Finance managers now work closely and are informed of every step. We changed the budgetary cycle to involve people at every stage.

Things are devolved through internal mechanisms but there are boundaries and limits so although it is devolved it is not completely let loose. It's like you are a dog in the garden you are chained to the post in some way. And I would say the culture of the organization right now allows people to do their own thing but within boundaries which aren't constraints, they are just boundaries which are set by the executive directors.

The new reduced directorate structure was reported as an attempt to strengthen lines of accountability to the centre. The trust was also in the process of reviewing its committee structure and setting out clear guidelines and terms of reference for each. An external report on the organization noted that the trust recognizes that there is still work to be done before these structures are fully embedded. In an effort to improve accountability and clinical performance a clinical scorecard system was being developed and was being used to gather information at departmental level about clinical activity and performance, including outpatient referral rates, contract monitoring data, waiting list and waiting times figures, cancelled operations, delayed discharges and A&E trolley waits. Establishing robust information systems was viewed as vital to the policy of devolving power down to clinical directorate level.

There was a feeling by some of those interviewed that the trust had managed to nurture more of a no blame culture under the new regime. However, others believed that problems still persisted and one person suggested that some of the trust's difficulties were due to its new openness in reporting external performance data:

> I think there is a no blame culture, and if you were to speak to nurses they would definitely say there is a difference from five years ago.

> I think nurses take responsibility for initiating and implementing a reporting policy ... We had an example recently where the students expressed concerns over the quality of nursing. And the students' voices were heard and an investigation is taking place right now. And I think we've got the right processes in place where students can say they've got a concern and an investigation happens because of that.

> There are still far too many instances where staff have not, for whatever reason, felt free to report incidents.

> I think we came a cropper on the star ratings because we were reporting accurately and not indulging in all the shenanigans. What you see is what you get. The current top team are very open and straightforward – if you've got problems you tell people about it.

Specific levers identified to help change the culture in the trust included the useful intervention of outside agencies such as CHI and work in relation to building up the professional confidence of nurses through education and training in order to challenge the traditional medical hierarchy in the trust:

> The [external evaluation] visit was a very helpful, positive experience for us as it endorsed a lot of the messages we were aware of . . . Our approach was 'great this is what we need, we are going to tell them exactly as it is because we need these people's help'. So we were full and frank and at pains to discuss the problems and difficulties that we had.

> We are trying to engender a sense of self-worth and confidence in the nursing staff. In a teaching hospital there is a hierarchy with the consultant on top and this has to be challenged if cultures are to change.

Staff reported a number of problems associated with recent changes in the organization. These centred on the increased pressures associated with having to meet demanding external targets and the re-direction of resources towards areas that are measured in the star rating system to the exclusion of other areas of clinical activity:

> I think a lot of people, general managers, nurses, have to work under a lot of pressure and strain here. In terms of having to meet the targets, whether they are achievable or not puts people under a lot of pressure.

> There are many pressures and we will have a very difficult year. It wears everyone down trying to meet the targets.

> Lots more emphasis on the performance indicators and how to meet them . . . if we don't meet them, and I'd say it is impossible to meet them all and stay sane there is a lot of harsh words and the like targeted at the culprits – even if it really is not their fault at all.

> Well I manage [name of directorate] and apart from our contribution to the electives, we don't really impact on the star system. So it feels that a lot of the time what we do as a directorate is not important to them because

we are not starred. It doesn't get resources directed at it, not because it is not a high quality service.

Concluding remarks

Many of Trust D's performance problems stemmed from the virtual sequestration of the senior management team from the wider organization. In particular senior clinicians and middle managers were excluded from participation in key corporate decisions and therefore all the considerations around service planning and financing were not considered fully. The large number of clinical directorates also seems to have hampered performance management in the trust. The new chief executive has sought to address this problem by reducing the number of clinical directorates and was focusing attention on improving lines of accountability within the organization. However staff reported the new attention paid to performance management was creating an uncomfortable climate for some staff because of the increased pressures associated with meeting externally driven performance targets.

TRUST E   LEARNING TO LET GO

The Trust is a large district general hospital which was awarded three stars in the performance ratings. The organization had a stable senior management team and the chief executive had been in post for many years.

Style of leadership and management orientation

Many of the senior management team at Trust E had a long association with the trust and this, it was stated, helped to engender a common purpose and direction in policy. The dominant style of leadership at the trust was described as largely top-down and transactional with a strong focus on meeting external performance targets, although there was a belief by some that this was evolving into a more participatory style of management (discussed below). The strong performance culture nurtured in the trust had also been highlighted in an external report on the organization. Staff talked with pride of a strong 'can do' culture at the trust and the cultural taboos were said to be not hitting performance targets or stating that something could not be done:

> I am personally performance oriented [chief executive speaking]. We should be setting ourselves targets, setting ourselves goals, and part of those goals is to be in the top 10 percent of any performance indicator that is around. That is our target.

> I think, by and large, the corporate priorities are driven by the star rating indicators. We do try and look at all areas of our performance but, when push comes to shove, we have to meet the external ones first otherwise we are under threat of losing stars which is in no one's best interests. Most people seem to be on board with that philosophy which helps us to all work together to make sure we hit these targets.

> My targets [chief executive speaking] come from two things. They come from our business planning process which starts at directorate level, the directorates being asked about their three year plans and priorities. And secondly from national targets.

> We have a distinct culture, at least compared within our peer group around here. For some time we have realized the benefits of focusing on performance. Clearly defined targets that people are expected to achieve. Some of which are driven nationally, some of which are imposed ourselves.

> You never say you can't do something. You find an answer no matter how difficult it is to do . . . that's encouraged here and if you don't like it well you know what you can do.

When external people come to [name of trust] one of
the first things they say is 'we are a performance driven
organization'. Now I take it for granted that where
there is a national indicator we will hit those targets.

It was reported the present strong performance orientated
culture in the organization was rooted in the vision of the
chief executive (and to a lesser extent the rest of the senior
management team) when he set up the trust. In particular
the chief executive was viewed as instrumental in developing
and embedding the internal systems and processes required,
creating and maintaining a high performance organization.
He was also widely believed to possess the personal qualities
required to challenge entrenched professional power bases,
especially the powerful consultant body that had previously
exerted a strong influence over policies in the organization:

I think it started [the origins of the performance cul-
ture] at the very top – I think the chief executive and
the executive team at the trust's inception – with what
sort of organization they would like to be leading. I
suspect it was very much a top-down starting point.

When I came in [chief executive speaking] it was run by
a medical mafia that saw themselves as operating outside normal employer/employee relationships. That
still goes on in the majority of NHS hospitals. And we
set about changing that.

There had been recent attempts to shift away from a
purely top-down transactional style of management
towards developing more of an inclusive and participatory
model. It was reported that were numerous initiatives being
developed to devolve power and responsibility down to clinical directorates and clinical teams when they had demonstrated a willingness and ability and take on such freedoms:

It is still very much about objective setting and we see
that in performance reviews, in objective setting for the
executive and divisional teams which is cascaded down

to clinical directors and business managers. So there is much objective setting. But personally I think we are seeing a change in style in that we are encouraging more freedom wherever possible.

I am happy to see the Stalinist control culture changing to a more hands off approach ... but I also see the dangers of doing that. Now giving freedom to people also means you have to be prepared to let them fail as well.

I think it is very difficult when you are performing to such a high standard, which we are, to let go of the reigns. But the other side is if you do not let go and let people innovate you're probably not going to hit your targets and maintain your performance.

Our performance management type culture is: You've got the freedom, you've got responsibility to manage your affairs but we're going to be looking over your shoulder to make sure you're not letting us down. If it moves we measure it. If it doesn't we want to know why.

The targets are not centrally driven. What we have done is work with the directorates and say these are the national imperatives and we agree a prioritization plan.

The chief executive is a very challenging and strategic figure and a strong leader. But is certainly prepared to develop the skills of clinical staff. He is extremely keen to hear what the views of forward thinking clinicians are. I think this has been the key to some of our success. The culture and the idea of using performance information and target setting has been very much driven by the chief exec and engaging clinical staff has helped to deliver that. If you didn't engage clinical directors then there is no doubt we wouldn't deliver.

It would appear that this shift towards a more participatory culture was triggered, at least in part, by criticism of an external report which noted that there were perceived problems that had arisen because of the autocratic and directive management style at the trust. In particular it noted that:

- Some senior clinicians reported that the directive style of senior management had led to feelings of lack of inclusivity and disempowerment, attributed to a lack of effective communication with or involvement of clinicians in service planning.
- There was evidence of a lack of two-way communication between frontline clinical staff and senior managers over key risk management issues.
- Staff expressed strong concerns about the high performance expectations aimed at senior managers (particularly business managers) and a lack of support when these expectations cannot be met.

Accountability and use of information

Trust E had strong and clear lines of accountability. Each of the senior executive team had a well-defined area of responsibility, particularly in relation to those aspects of the trust's activity that were externally monitored. A senior clinician had been appointed as head of performance, and to co-ordinate trust-wide activities around delivering the performance management agenda. Monitoring and accountability arrangements for performance and clinical governance included regularly scheduled meetings at all levels of the hierarchy. The performance manager within each directorate met with each business manager and clinical director on a monthly basis to discuss and report on performance issues:

> Accountability structures here are very well-defined and in the open for all to see. Everyone from the chief executive downwards to the junior nurses are fully aware of what is expected of them and their role in helping us to improve . . . So there really is nowhere for people to hide if you screw up, and no one else to blame if you do.

> The vision is very clear in the organization. People might not understand the detailed plans but everyone

knows it is around the putting patients first and excellence in health care.

A huge amount in terms of clarity of vision, purpose and the ability to communicate that, is down to [the chief executive] – and within that everyone knows what is expected of them here.

It was reported that the trust had very good information systems and senior managers had decided to invest in developing robust reporting and monitoring arrangements to support performance management. The CHI clinical governance report noted that the availability and use of clinical information was an area of good practice within the trust. National clinical indicators and health outcomes are continuously monitored and reported routinely. The trust adopted a proactive approach to developing information databases to support performance management. For example, areas of performance that may be subject to external performance monitoring in the future are anticipated in advance and monitored using 'shadow performance indicators' which allow the trust to assess how to develop its information systems and to highlight any possible problems meeting these targets:

And we have tried to design a structure that focuses our clinical directorates and their teams on performance, supported by the right quality data, which we've invested in quite heavily. That ensures that we monitor and track performance and staff are aware of how they are doing against defined standards.

The key driver at this trust is devolving as much as possible to frontline staff ... We give a directorate a budget. But if you are going to give people budgetary control you've got to have a good mechanism for monitoring what they are doing because that clearly puts the organization at risk.

It is part of my job to maintain our internal performance indicators in line with what is the national direction. So we review our indicators every year to ensure that all the important external ones are incorporated internally.

If there is an indicator that is coming up 12 months or two years down the line we would try to anticipate that by shadow monitoring. So that at least we are used to collecting the information, and reporting it and have some idea how we are performing.

Learning and reflexive practice

Trust E was working to develop a no blame policy on clinical incidence reporting and near misses. Many staff also talked of creating more of an open culture at the organization where staff could feel free to report and learn from mistakes. Some staff, however, thought that the trust had a considerable way to go before staff would feel safe to report problems, given the strong performance management culture at the trust. Indeed, an external report on the organization noted that although there were a number of good examples of learning from incidents and near misses, there was compelling evidence to suggest that serious incidents had not been reported, either because of a lack of understanding of the process or a lack of recognition of the importance of the process:

> We are honest as an organization and with staff. We are very clear about when we think we are good, but we are also very clear about the bad. So we'll sing our praises to the sky but we'll also say we are crap at this or that.

> Incident reporting is an area we have struggled to get to grips with. I think it is one of the weaknesses in the organization.

> We have an ethos here that strives for the best and excellence all the time . . . when something happens which threatens this it is often uncomfortable for the person concerned and there may be an issue around

how much people are willing to report mistakes and learn from them . . . as an organization we never like to acknowledge that we're not the best.

External relationships

Trust E adopted a very proactive approach towards developing close relationships with key external stakeholders and organizations within the local health economy. It was recognized that meeting many of the key government performance targets, especially those around waiting times and readmission rates depended on a 'whole systems approach' to managing the local health economy. Indeed, an external report applauded the trust for the steps it had taken to establish a panel comprising key members of patient advocacy organizations and patient and service user representatives:

> I think we are doing some very good work around how we work with partners, how we change services, how we interact with the whole system and secure change.

> It is your job to understand how other systems work [chief executive speaking]. I've never worked in social services and yet it is important for me to understand and influence social services. We fought like cat and dog over some things but both organizations deliver and that's been really helpful . . . The weak player has been the health authority and primary care.

> Some of the partner organizations in the area are not well developed in terms of their performance management arrangements and how well they deliver. I think one of the single most important hindrances is our primary care set up. We are not well provided for in terms of high quality primary care and that puts added pressure on emergency services in secondary care.

> We have been saying for some time that management of the waiting lists is not a secondary care problem. It is a joint primary/secondary care problem. And the people who can influence it most are primary care.

Human resource policies

It was reported that Trust E placed great emphasis on developing and harnessing the potential of staff to deliver the performance improvement agenda. An external report on the organization noted that the trust had demonstrated a clear commitment to staff education and training. It recognized that these programmes are well connected to the needs of the organization and that there are clearly established systems of identifying and meeting training needs. From the interviews and supporting documentation it was clear that the trust places considerable emphasis on the recruitment and retention of staff that are considered compatible with a high performance environment. Indeed, the trust had invested heavily in development of courses for consultants and new staff to 'enculture' the right attitude and behaviour:

> We invested quite heavily in training and education of our clinical directors and the general consultant body, some might say this was conditioning to say look these are the rules of the game. This is the environment we play in. This is what we are trying to do, we want you to learn to manage budgets, to learn how to manage people, to deliver on targets.

> When setting up the organization we put quite a lot of money into organizational development. At the start around clinical directors but now every consultant has run through some form of OD at least once if not twice.

> It is OK having a very focused set of performance indicators and setting targets for the organization . . . It's actually about what you do to get the change to actually deliver those targets . . . how do you get the behavioural and cultural change.

> We are very clear about the sort of processes which should be in place but it is all centred around the patient to make sure the patient gets the best deal. And we can only give the patient the best deal by

developing our own staff. By developing our own staff that they are skilled, equipped, up to date, motivated, etc. they will provide the best patient care possible.

At one of the recent consultant interviews we failed to appoint. We've done that at least three times over the last couple of years where we have had candidates and failed to appoint – despite chronic shortages. That was when candidates did not convince us at interview that they had the right skills we wanted. So it is based on personality traits and the like. Other trusts are less picky and may have much more trouble trying to manage those people later.

The strong performance orientated culture of the organization was associated with exemplary performance on many of the nationally set indicators. However some staff reported that it did cause problems not necessarily picked up by external assessments. These included the fact that the emphasis on meeting national targets sometimes distorted clinical priorities and the provision of high quality patient care; the stress and heavy workload staff had to labour under caused by the 'excessively' high expectations and demands placed on staff by some senior managers; and feelings that because the trust was such a high performing organization it often did not benefit from the advice and expertise of external organizations such as the Modernisation Agency:

The two-week outpatient cancer wait. In terms of my clinical experience and managerial experience this is not a sensible target in that there is no great added value for patients in seeing them within that time frame. So the indicator is not a good indicator of patient outcomes because it probably doesn't influence patient outcomes that much. However, it is the national indicator so we will choose to hit that target.

We are driven more and more by central targets and being a high performing trust we are often asked for for what would be more sensible in terms of the performance management framework for the NHS. And our message is fewer targets and if possible more clinician driven, sensible targets. Targets based on outcomes rather than processes.

The stresses and strains of working in an organization can be very high that is the downside . . . I'm sure some really feel that especially when we are pushing for delivery on a target.

We are high performing but sometimes that works against you because we don't get as much help as we would like from all the external agencies because they think we are all right thank you very much. They focus their efforts on the ones that have been deemed poor.

Concluding remarks

Trust E has a strong performance driven culture. The dominant style of leadership was transactional with a focus on meeting external performance targets, although there were signs that this was slowly evolving into more devolved and participatory styles of management. The trust was characterized by a strong 'can do' culture with the ultimate taboo described as not meeting external performance targets. Considerable emphasis was placed on recruiting staff whose personalities and skills fitted the high performance culture of the organization. Attention was also focused on promoting a corporate ethos amongst clinicians, and other professional groups, through a range of human resources initiatives, including specialized training and staff development programmes.

However, staff did report that the strong performance management culture of the organization sometimes caused problems that were not picked up by the national performance indicators or formal assessments by external agencies. For example, the emphasis on meeting national performance targets was reported to have distorted some clinical priorities and on occasions militated against the provision of high quality patient care. In addition, the very high performance expectations placed on staff at all levels of the hierarchy was said to generate a very heavy workload and in some cases cause excessive stress and anxiety amongst managers.

TRUST F 'CAN DO' TEAM

Trust F provides the majority of district general hospital services and was awarded three stars in the performance ratings. A key emergent theme from this case study is the emphasis placed on using human resources policies to develop and harness the potential of staff to deliver the external performance management agenda.

Leadership style and management orientation

The trust has a very stable management team, and although it has recently had a change of chief executive, the person appointed was one of the previous executive directors and there had been few changes at executive director level over the preceding five years. The stability of the senior management team was said to be a good platform for creating a high performance organization:

> I think that we've had quite a lot of stability as an organization and over the last five years a lot of organizations have not had that stability and it does make a difference. I think internal stability is important in two respects. First of all it's important because it creates clarity of approach, clarity of values and principles that people know. It also helps to feel more in control because there is a constant framework.

> The executive here have been very stable. Since we've become a trust we have only had two changes of executive director which I think is unusual. One was the medical director and we appointed a clinical who was

here to that. So we have had a very stable top team which allows you to think of things in the longer term. I think that goes for the next tier down as well and we've had a very stable clinical directorate structure with senior managers.

I think the management structure is sound in as much as the clinical directorates are led by clinicians who have a strong interest in management and who have got a lot of management experience. So it is a fairly stable management structure in that respect.

We don't have a specific strategy [culture change] it's an organic thing. Because the executive team is broadly stable a culture has evolved around ways of doing things here that you couldn't probably design and implement but it is the organic product of a large number of different factors.

The current chief executive, like his predecessor, was described as pursuing a balance of transactional and trans-formational approaches to managing the trust. Thus it was reported that the centre set a strong strategic direction for the trust with clear messages and targets for staff and clinical directorates. However, a high degree of responsibility had been devolved to individual clinical directorates who had considerable freedoms and discretion over how to allocate resources and design services around the needs of patients. Ordinarily the senior management team only became involved in operational details when a clinical directorate or individual service area were under-performing. In many respects the senior management culture appeared to reflect many of the values underpinning the policy of earned autonomy as set out in the NHS plan, because considerable power was devolved down to the frontline staff with the centre intervening only if performance was not up to standard:

The overwhelming majority of resources are down at clinical directorate level. We are talking about 80 percent plus of resources.

An aspect of the culture is decentralization – devolving both financial and other powers and authority so that people can manage close to the frontline – and I think directorates have developed like that over the years. But while there has been decentralization there has also been a clear steer from the executives as a team as to what needs doing and the priorities. So there is a very centrally determined approach to performance management.

We have a sort of rapid response culture within the organization so if they are over 13 week waiters at the end of September then I guarantee a meeting will be held with the clinical director about what he's going to do before the end of November. So there is an immediate response.

There was a strong performance management culture at the Trust and considerable emphasis was placed at all levels of the hierarchy on meeting external performance targets. Staff commonly referred to a 'can do' culture at the trust. Senior staff were not always in agreement with the external performance targets but they viewed meeting them as a 'necessary evil' in order to provide enough space for meeting locally determined priorities:

The most telling feel for the place is that we've developed an all embracing culture of internal performance management. This covers everything that can be nailed down and measured. If it can't be measured we develop a way of doing it.

I think this organization is as good as it gets in terms of focusing on the 'must be dones'. It is good on performance management. We are obsessed with targets and, I'll be perfectly honest, that is not necessarily because we wholeheartedly support some of the targets, because we don't; but we will sign up to them.

I think we have a legitimate representation as a 'can do' approach . . . It is said without prompting. I've heard a number of managers separately say it on a number of occasions and I think it is something that has organically developed. It's not something that you can say 'right we're going to be a can-do organization' it's something that evolves.

We have a . . . 'can do' culture – so if you give us a set of standards and a task then we are very good at doing those things.

I think part of the culture here is this continuously competitive thing, striving for excellence.

The vast majority of the NHS [targets] nobody has a problem with. But there are one or two areas which I think we are less enthusiastic about and I think there are some areas which are wrong if I am honest. But there is absolutely no point in head butting a national target. So the attitude we've engendered on this site is let's get compliance. Let's deliver the must-be-dones and then we can do the want-to-dos.

Our main reason for trying to meet external targets is that you tend to be left alone so that you can maximize scope to manage your services and deliver services in a way which you feel appropriate.

Although senior staff espoused a vision to create a devolved, participatory style of management, some of the senior clinicians reported that the strong central emphasis on performance management sometimes militated against their close involvement in setting the corporate agenda. Yet other staff did report that there was a strong sense of informality at the organization and a distinct lack of hierarchy. This may in part be explained by the fact that senior staff perceived that there was a lack of hierarchy but staff lower down the organization were certainly aware of top-down management, especially when national performance targets were in danger of not being achieved:

I would say it is very centrally driven. The amount of work that is going to be delivered is very much dictated from above and there is perhaps not quite as much discussion with clinicians in deciding what is deliverable.

There is a large degree of informality and the absence of a conscious sense of hierarchy. Most people are on first name terms, we don't stand on ceremony. The senior managers don't spend a lot of time reminding people what their status is.

They [the senior management team] are not that interventionist with my team but that's because we've delivered on everything that has been asked of us . . . I know for a fact and other colleagues who've experienced this is, that they'd come down like a ton of bricks if we didn't.

Accountability and use of information

Trust F had very strong and transparent lines of accountability with all senior staff having clear lines of responsibility for areas of measured performance. Considerable resources had been directed at developing robust information systems for monitoring financial and clinical performance. The high degree of devolution in the trust was made possible by the quality of information that could be used by the centre to monitor the performance of clinical directorates:

I think the corporate infrastructure is there. We have structured ourselves corporately so that we have a robust way of understanding what's happening and monitoring it.

I feel it is a need within my directorate to meet the targets. I regard it as a priority because I don't want to let the team down. I'm part of the team. I'm part of the management. And I have to do my bit to try and ensure that we do meet the target and we take it personally if we fall down.

I think one of the reasons that we succeed and I believe other organizations perform well is by concentrating on the basics. It is a question of making sure the basic systems and processes work, that day-to-day services are properly delivered. A lot of organizations focus on the strategy without getting the basics rights. Do they know what is going on in the organization and can they measure it properly.

Human resources policies

There was considerable emphasis on staff development and training at Trust F. In particular attention was focused on developing a corporate ethos amongst clinical staff and encouraging clinicians to take on management responsibilities. The organization was very discriminating in its recruitment of clinical staff and great store was placed on attracting and retaining staff with the required 'can do' mentality. This situation was said to be made all the more easier because the trust had a very high reputation amongst clinicians and the high star rating classification had enhanced the trust's reputation still further. The relatively young cohort of consultants at the trust made culture change easier, as these people were more inclined to seek and take up corporate management responsibilities than their older colleagues:

> We tend to have the choice over medical staff.

> In the interviews over the last five years or so I can remember recruiting for a number of senior management posts and the questions about 'can do' are always cropping up at the forefront of the interview. You are always looking for people who are striving for excellence.

> Our priority when we make appointments has been to say 'how will this person work within our organization and within our department?' I would call it a cultural policy. I would say that has been the strongest cultural policy running through the department on recent years.

A lot of work and resources have been spent on education and training strategies.

We have good training and educational programmes and that has helped to attract the right calibre of clinical staff.

The average age of the consultant medical staff is very young for a hospital this size. We are having one or two retirements each year which is a small number. I think it gives a distinctive culture because there's less inheritance from a historical culture. The benefit of having a relatively young senior staff and medical staff is that they are less set in their ways and open to change. They are more challenging and less prepared to accept the status quo.

The place got a buzz out of being a three star because everyone wanted to work in what was perceived to be the best organization. Everyone wants to play for [a Premiership club], no one wants to work for [a lower division club] – you know it's just a fact of life.

External relationships

Trust F was reported to have relatively good relationships with other key organizations in the local economy. In order to ensure that there was a health community overview for clinical governance and to reduce the risk of repetition of effort a specific group was established to work in this area. In addition:

We are very active in forging good relationships with all the local health agencies and social services. We try and set and lead the local agenda. That way we can deliver a more seamless service for patients.

With social services we've got a good history. We've been around a long time so we've established good working relationships. I think the relationships are pretty good. We have excellent relationships with GPs.

Dysfunctional consequences

A number of dysfunctional effects of the culture change agenda at Trust F were identified. These mainly related to a distortion in clinical priorities caused by the national performance indicators. Barriers to culture change identified in the trust related to changing entrenched professional practices and the diversity of cultures within the organization which made it difficult to implement a common approach to levering change:

> [Chief executive speaking] The only area we were not very clever on [was star rating indicators]. This year some initial money was put out for cancelled operations and the three starred trusts got less than all the others. I got less on the area I needed to improve on. So I was more than pissed off about that. The second disbenefit of being a three starred trust is that we were told that our proposals for action on initiative money would go straight to the Department of Health. It did and we got nothing and I know for a fact that if it had gone through our regional office ours would have been a high priority.

> The one area we accept what we've got to do better on cancer waits. Then the league table comes out and we get less money than everyone else and people are saying to me in the corridor 'Shouldn't we be two star next year if the money's coming out on that basis'.

> It has given me some problems because one or two areas have said 'if you want to be a three star make sure you need to sort this out. So there's been some blatant blackmail. 'If you want trolley waits down then we need an extra porter.'

> In Community Children's Services you have doctors, including consultants, who are part of a multidisciplinary team looking after children with complex problems and the performance targets say that everyone has to be seen within 13 weeks. It's 13 weeks for

those children who are referred to by a doctor or GP, but into that same clinical service there may be educationalists who will refer a child in, there may be other professions, physiotherapists, speech therapists who will refer children. Yet we are on a 13-week wait for that isolated group who are referred to by doctors. Who are no different from any of the others and we have no choice but to concentrate on those and potentially downgrade some clinical priorities to make sure we meet those targets.

Some, though far from all, of the clinicians are reluctant to embrace the modernizing movement and prefer to retreat into their professional worlds when challenged. They are the hardest to shift but this organization has a good record on making them move towards a more acceptable working practice.

The barriers are the fact that you have a number of different types of workplace, each of which tends to have its own culture. You've got office environments, you've got the factory elements, e.g. sterilization and disinfection unit, and then you've got the unique environments of health care wards and operating theatres. And although it's a single organization there are a lot of cultures to manage.

Concluding remarks

Trust F had developed a strong 'can do' culture and a stable management team had placed an emphasis on establishing robust internal reporting systems to support the external performance management agenda. The organization was developing a devolved system of management, which was facilitated, in part, by the strong lines of accountability and good information system that had been established within the organization. A particular performance related feature was the importance the organization placed on developing a human resources strategy that would support its high performance ambitions. The organization was placing a high priority on recruiting and retaining staff who displayed a commitment to following the corporate rather than a purely professional agenda. It was also adopting a proactive approach to managing the local health economy. However the emphasis on meeting performance targets was reported to have distorted clinical priorities in the organization.

In the following chapter we broaden our analysis and report the findings of a national quantitative study which teamed a validated culture rating instrument with a comprehensive performance database to assess the relationship between senior management team culture and performance in NHS acute hospital trusts. The intention was to see to what extent the culture/performance patterns seen in our six case studies might be repeated nationally.

5

FINDINGS FROM A QUANTITATIVE ANALYSIS OF ALL ENGLISH NHS ACUTE TRUSTS
(with Rowena Jacobs)

The acute trust case studies reported in the two previous chapters provided compelling evidence for the importance of culture in shaping performance within hospitals. The additional piece of empirical work reported in this chapter builds on this by exploring culture/performance relationships quantitatively in a much wider group of NHS hospitals. We report measured associations between NHS acute trust senior management team culture and various routinely collected measures of organizational characteristics and performance. This work was carried out across *all* English NHS acute trusts and is used to complement and broaden the case study analyses already presented.

AIMS

The work sought to explore three key ideas. First, can senior management team culture in the NHS acute sector be assessed? Second, is senior management team culture related to organizational characteristics and performance? And third, what is the evidence that any such relationships are contingent? Each of these draws on both the conceptual understanding of culture developed in Chapter 1 and the experience of previous empirical studies outlined and discussed in Chapter 2. Findings from this broader analysis were also used to triangulate the complementary findings arising from the acute trust case studies presented in previous chapters.

The analysis focused on all English NHS acute trusts. Notwithstanding recent and ongoing structural change (especially merger activity, Fulop *et al.* 2002), NHS acute trusts have clear organizational boundaries and (relatively) established identities. There is also a wide variety of performance data available on these entities, in particular composite ratings of performance in the form of the star rating system.

The three main study objectives are now expanded in turn:

- *Can senior management team culture in the NHS acute sector be assessed?* Relatively few studies have been conducted which have assessed senior management team culture in the NHS (Gerowitz *et al.* 1996; Scott *et al.* 2003c). One established instrument, the competing values framework (CVF) questionnaire (see later) has received extensive use in culture studies in the USA (e.g. Shortell *et al.* 2000), and we wanted to assess its practicability and usefulness as a tool for UK use. Thus the intention was to provide an account of the cultural landscape of the acute sector NHS trusts at senior management level.

- *Is senior management team culture related to organizational characteristics and performance?* This consists of exploratory work in two main areas. First, an examination of the trust characteristics that are associated with different cultural types as expressed by senior management and second, an exploration of any cross-sectional associations between different culture measures and various macro-level trust performance measures. We have only tentative prior hypotheses in this area, partly because we have only limited knowledge of likely relationships (these being relatively unexplored to date) and partly because any relationships are likely to be complex and contingent.

- *What is the evidence that any relationships between culture and performance are contingent?* Previous empirical work (e.g. Gerowitz *et al.* 1996), and our reading of the theoretical literature suggest that any relationship between culture and performance is unlikely to be simple. It seems more plausible that specific aspects of performance will be enhanced in cultures whose assumptions, beliefs and values underpin successful delivery in that area. We make some provisional suggestions as to what such contingent relationships might look like (see Table 5.1) and test these relationships in our data set.

The rest of this section proceeds as follows. We first explain the way in which senior management team culture was assessed in the acute trusts and outline the underlying structure of the competing values framework. Some tentative hypotheses are suggested concerning contingent relationships between trust culture and trust performance. We then go on to present the culture data, first on individuals, and then aggregating across individuals, calculating culture variables at trust level. Regression modelling (Model 1) is then used to explore the influence of job title, with adjusted data for the distribution of trust culture variables being presented.

Subsequent sections present the findings from a series of models linking culture to trust characteristics. These begin with simple correlations (Model 2) and ANOVA (Model 3), before using multinomial logit (Model 4) and ordered probit (Model 5) as a means of examining specifically the relationships between culture and performance. Detailed model specifications and findings are presented in Appendix 2, with the chapter narrative highlighting instead the key messages and their interpretation.

ASSESSING ORGANIZATIONAL CULTURE

Following a review of available instruments (Scott *et al.* 2003d) we decided to use the competing values framework, with some minor amendments made by Shortell and colleagues (who adapted it for a US health care setting: Shortell *et al.* 2000, 2001) and by ourselves (to convert it for use in the UK). We chose the CVF for the following reasons:

- Unlike most other available instruments, the CVF has a sound theoretical basis and attempts to address shared values as well as the more superficial manifestations of culture.
- The CVF has been used extensively in the UK and the USA in both health care and non-health care settings. As a result, whilst there is limited published evidence about its scientific properties, we are starting to understand more about how it can be used and what the results might mean.
- The questionnaire has strong face validity, is easy and quick to complete and has achieved acceptable response rates in other studies.
- As a global culture measurement instrument, the CVF is applicable in both the acute and primary care sectors and has proved to be acceptable to a range of staff groups.
- Because the CVF produces a culture typology, it is useful not only as a quantitative tool, but also as an explanatory framework to aid qualitative data analysis.

Box 5.1   Competing values model of culture types for organizations

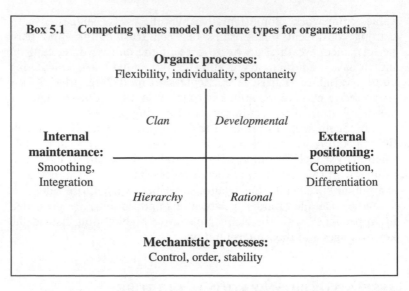

Application of the CVF leads to four culture types produced by a model based on two intersecting axes (see Box 5.1). The first axis relates to the processes that go on within an organization. At one extreme are the so-called 'organic processes' characterized by flexibility, individuality and spontaneity. At the other end are the so-called 'mechanistic processes', characterized by control, order and stability. The second axis relates to the positioning of the organization in relation to the outside world. At one end of the axis is so-called 'external positioning', characterized by competition and attempts at differentiation. At the other end is 'internal maintenance', characterized by smoothing activities and integration.

Internally focused organizations using organic processes are described as having a 'clan' culture, whilst internally focused organizations using mechanistic processes are described as having a 'hierarchical' culture. Outward-looking organizations using organic processes are referred to as having a 'developmental' culture, whilst outward-looking organizations using mechanistic processes are referred to as having a 'rational' culture. The key characteristics of these four culture types, in terms of the cultural attributes, leadership style, the 'glue' that holds the staff together and the strategic emphasis of the organization are described in Box 5.2.

The CVF is operationalized through use of a self-completed questionnaire. The questionnaire offers respondents a series of

Box 5.2   **Characteristics of culture types in the competing values framework**

Clan:	Developmental:
cohesive, participative	creative, adaptive
leader as mentor	leader as risk-taker, innovator
bonded by loyalty, tradition	bonded by entrepreneurship
emphasis on morale	emphasis on innovation
Hierarchical:	**Rational:**
order, rules, uniformity	competitiveness
leader as administrator	leader as goal-oriented
bonded by rules, policies	bonded by competition
emphasis on predictability	emphasis on winning

descriptions of a hospital, arranged in five groups of four. Within each group of four descriptions, the respondent is asked to 'share 100 points' between them 'according to which description best fits your current organization'. The five groups represent descriptions of hospital characteristics, leadership, emphasis, cohesion and rewards. Collating these points allocations provides a score (in the range 0–100) for each individual on each of four cultural subtypes: clan, developmental, hierarchical or rational.

The largest score on each cultural subtype defines that individual's *dominant culture type*; the actual value of this score represents the *strength* of that dominant cultural type. The sum of the scores for clan and hierarchy gives the cultural *focus* (internal versus external); the sum of the scores for clan and developmental gives the cultural *orientation* (relational versus mechanistic). The dominant culture type, strength, focus and orientation for an organization (in this case an NHS acute trust) are calculated by aggregating across the individual scores of the senior management team in that organization.

Boxes 5.1 and 5.2 show the underlying value structure of the competing values framework. Thus, organizations are seen to be in tension between the four underlying culture types, with their scores representing the extent of that tension.

Hypothesized relationships between cultural types and aspects of performance

An understanding of the values, beliefs and assumptions that underpin the competing values framework (Boxes 5.1 and 5.2) allows a number of hypotheses to be derived about any relationship between culture and performance. If a contingency view is correct, then those aspects of performance valued within a given culture should be those aspects of performance that are enhanced in trusts that exhibit strong congruence with that culture. Some such hypotheses are shown in Table 5.1.

Individual data on organizational culture

Requests for completion of the CVF were sent to the senior management team (Trust Board) for 197 trusts in England. Of 1508 questionnaires mailed, usable responses were received from 899 individuals, a base response rate of 60 percent. In assessing the trusts' culture we are seeking robust estimates of senior management views, and previous studies have usually regarded three or four key senior managers' responses as sufficient to define the organizational culture type (Gerowitz *et al.* 1996; Gerowitz 1998). In this study, at least one senior manager responded from 189 of the 197 trusts (96 percent); at least three senior managers responded from 170 trusts (86 percent); and four or more replied from 145 (74 percent), hence we attained excellent coverage of English acute trusts.

Quality of completion of the questionnaire was very high. Each culture assessment question was completed by over 98 percent of respondents, and only 2 to 3 percent of these responses required minor arithmetical adjustment. (Respondents were asked to share 100 points between four statements, but sometimes this share out summed to more or less than 100. In such discrepant cases the numbers were adjusted proportionally to force a sum to 100.)

In responding to the culture assessment questions, respondents provided highly variable responses (standard deviations for each culture type were 10–14) using almost the full range of responses available (see Table 5.2). Clan culture scored the highest overall mean (31), followed by rational culture (mean 27). Thus the majority of individuals fell into clan as their dominant culture (47 percent), followed by rational (23 percent). The mean culture strength was 41.

In terms of distinguishing internal versus external focus, and mechanistic versus relational orientation, the scores are shown in

Table 5.1   Contingent performance: hypothesized relationships

	Valued aspects	*Expected performance variables favoured*
Dominant culture type		
Clan	Tradition, cohesion, commitment, morale. Internal culture focus and relational cultural orientation.	Staffing levels, staff opinions/morale, higher degree of specialization, higher level of cancelled ops, high trust, named doctor/nurse; may have poorer star ratings.
Developmental	Innovation, dynamism, growth, entrepreneurship. External culture focus and relational cultural orientation.	Waiting times; Better star ratings.
Hierarchical	Order, procedures, stability, predictability. Internal culture focus and mechanistic cultural orientation.	Data quality, financial balance – but perhaps higher costs associated with bureaucracy.
Rational	External competitiveness, achievement. External culture focus and mechanistic cultural orientation.	Research revenue, costs; Better star ratings.
Cultural orientation:		
Mechanistic	Rationality, rules, ordered decision making.	Measures of conformity.
Relational	Interpersonal, bonded, shared experience.	Staff morale.
Culture focus:		
Internal	Maintaining the internal organizational integrity.	Staff morale, staffing levels.
External	Engaging with the external environment.	Waiting times, star ratings and other formal performance indicators, low level complaints, rapidly dealt with.

Table 5.2 Average culture scores for individuals across four culture types (n=899)

	Mean	Std Dev	Min	Max	Percentage of individuals with this as dominant culture type
Clan	30.96	14.06	0	86	46.7%
Developmental	23.04	10.92	0	100	16.7%
Hierarchical	18.88	12.18	0	80	13.7%
Rational	27.11	10.69	0	72	22.9%
Culture strength	*40.91*	*10.03*	*26*	*100*	

Table 5.3 Average internal and mechanistic scores for individuals (n=899)

	Mean	*Std Dev*	*Min*	*Max*
Internal	49.84	13.37	0	100
External	50.16	13.37	0	100
Mechanistic	45.99	16.63	0	100
Relational	54.01	16.63	0	100

Table 5.3. These simply add together the relevant average culture scores to form the new focus/orientation score. Individuals were fairly evenly divided between these two pairs of categorizations.

The questionnaire contained data on (self-reported) job title so it was possible to break down the distribution of culture type according to the managerial post held (Table 5.4). Trust chairs and trust chief executives seem to have a stronger tendency for identifying with clan culture – 67 percent and 60 percent respectively fell into this category; while finance directors and medical directors contained the largest proportions aligned with a 'rational' culture (about a quarter in each case). As there may potentially be something systematic about the way people in specific jobs respond to these questions this is tested at a later stage.

A similar analysis by job type was conducted for external versus internal focus, and for mechanistic versus relational orientation (Table 5.5). In each job group respondents were fairly evenly divided between the two categories. One notable deviation from this even split was that 60 per cent of both chief executives and trust chairs were identified as having a relational orientation compared to just 40 per cent being identified as having a mechanistic orientation (Table 5.5).

Table 5.4 Distribution of culture type by job title (n=899)

Job title	Number of respondents	Dominant culture type (%)			
		Clan	Develop.	Hierarch.	Rational
Chief executive	92	59.78	17.39	5.43	17.39
Director finance	110	46.36	16.36	10.91	26.36
Director nursing	141	51.77	17.02	10.64	20.57
Medical director	143	42.66	23.08	9.79	24.48
Trust chair	103	66.99	9.71	7.77	15.53
Director HR	102	42.16	12.75	19.61	25.49
Other	179	34.08	14.53	24.02	27.37
Not stated	29	29.41	23.53	17.65	29.41

Table 5.5 Cultural focus and orientation by job title (n=899)

Job title	Number of respondents	Culture focus (%)		Culture orientation (%)	
		Internal	External	Mechanistic	Relational
Chief executive	92	50.05	49.95	39.95	60.05
Director finance	110	49.40	50.60	47.24	52.76
Director nursing	141	50.05	49.95	43.32	56.68
Medical director	143	48.35	51.65	45.76	54.24
Trust chair	103	52.62	47.38	40.48	59.52
Director HR	102	50.78	49.22	48.85	51.15
Other	179	49.01	50.99	51.77	48.23
Not stated	29	48.94	51.06	46.90	53.10

Aggregating across individuals to assess the trust culture

Trust-level scores were computed by averaging the scores across all valid individual scores. This was done for each question and for each culture type with the dominant score then being taken across the trust as a whole. A variable (weight) was created to take account of the number of respondents per trust with the assumption that culture type derived from higher numbers of respondents per trust provides a more robust assessment. This weight was used in later regressions and with descriptive analyses, but was found in practice to have negligible effects.

DESCRIBING TRUST CULTURES

Descriptive data on culture for the final merged data set are given in both unweighted (Table 5.6) and weighted (Table 5.7) forms. As there is no substantive difference between these future analyses largely show unweighted scores (although both weighted and unweighted models were developed for confirmation). Trust score distributions across the four culture types (Tables 5.6 and 5.7) closely mirror the pattern seen in individual scores (Table 5.2), but with lower levels of variation. It is worth noting that all cultural types received significant scoring (indicating that values are indeed *competing*), from a mean of 19 (hierarchical) to a mean of 31 (clan). As expected, overall culture strength is also lower when calculated across trusts (mean 36.6) than when calculated at individual level (mean 40.9). Patterns of culture focus (internal/external) and culture orientation (external/internal) across trusts also mirrored those across individuals (Table 5.8: trust-level data and Table 5.3: individual-level data).

Table 5.6   Average culture scores for trusts across four culture types, unweighted (n=187)

	Mean	*Std Dev*	*Min*	*Max*
Clan	31.15	9.69	0	64
Developmental	22.71	7.29	3	49
Hierarchical	18.82	7.94	2	52
Rational	27.33	6.79	13	47
Culture strength	*36.61*	*6.11*	*27*	*64*

Table 5.7   Average culture scores for trusts across four culture types, weighted (n=187)

	Mean	*Std Dev*	*Min*	*Max*
Clan	30.94	8.99	0	64
Developmental	23.07	6.95	3	49
Hierarchical	18.82	7.10	2	52
Rational	27.17	6.37	13	47
Culture strength	*36.06*	*5.58*	*27*	*64*

Table 5.8 Average internal and mechanistic scores for trusts, unweighted (n=187)

	Mean	*Std Dev*	*Min*	*Max*
Internal	49.96	9.18	29	80
External	50.04	9.18	20	71
Mechanistic	46.14	11.25	19	97
Relational	53.86	11.25	3	81

Allocating trusts to dominant culture types was accomplished in the standard way of identifying the highest score. Over half of the trusts (54 percent) were identified as clan dominant culture type; 29 percent were rational, 11 percent developmental, and just 6 percent hierarchical (see Figure 5.1). Thus moving from *individual* assessments of culture type to *organizational* assessments saw more trusts (proportionally) as clan and rational and fewer as developmental or hierarchical (see the data on individuals in Table 5.2). It is also worth noting that this means of assigning 'dominant culture type' (by choosing the type with the largest value) accentuates the difference seen between mean scores assigned to each of the subtypes. Thus, whereas the average score across trusts for clan culture of 31 translated into 54 percent of trusts being assigned this as the dominant culture type, the average score for hierarchical culture of 19 translates into just 6 percent of trusts being assigned this as the dominant culture. Thus the culture typing approach can sometimes mask important tensions (i.e. competing values). For this reason, in the analysis we make use of both the dominant culture types allocated to trusts *and* their means scores on each of the separate culture subtypes.

Model 1: Adjusting for senior management role

It may be the case that the respondents' job role has a systematic effect on the way individuals respond to the questionnaire. Hence, regressions were run on the average scores for each individual culture subtype (clan, developmental, hierarchical, rational), controlling for their job title by a set of dummy variables based on their job code. Running a fixed effect model in each case, this effectively generates an individual hospital-specific score that may be considered the 'true' hospital culture score, purged of job title effects (see Model 1[1]).

The results from Model 1 suggest that potentially job titles 2 (director of finance), 6 (director of HR), 7 (director of quality) and

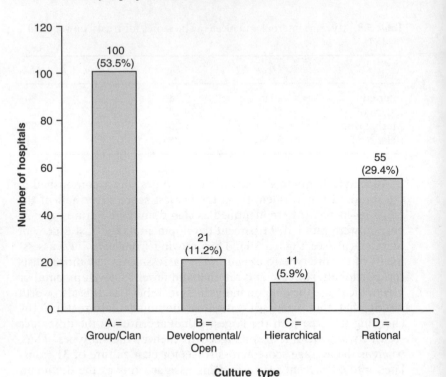

Figure 5.1 Frequency distribution of culture type by trusts, unweighted (n=187)

9 (other) are more likely to overstate hierarchical culture compared to clan culture. However, whilst adjusting for job title does appear to be important in determining culture type, further models (see later) have used the unadjusted culture scores in the first instance (although the results using these adjusted culture scores were also calculated they did not much influence the overall picture). This is because there may be other important individual characteristics that may influence respondents which we have not been able to account for and which may affect the results in either direction. Hence the unadjusted culture scores are to be preferred in the absence of any further rationale for additional adjustments.

RELATING TRUST CULTURE TO ORGANIZATIONAL CHARACTERISTICS AND PERFORMANCE

In the following sections the relationships are explored between culture scores/dominant cultures and various trust characteristics, including a range of performance measures (see data descriptions in Appendix 2). Descriptive analyses (correlations and analysis of variance) are used initially to explore these relationships, so that along with the *a priori* testable hypotheses, any relationships uncovered can inform the variable choices for further modelling.

Model 2: Correlations of trust culture variables with other trust variables

The first descriptive analysis explored the correlations of each of the four main culture variables with a host of other trust characteristics (for full details see Model 2, Appendix 2). Generally fairly low correlations were evidenced. However the scores for clan culture often showed moderate *negative* correlations (<−0.3) with a wide range of trust measures. In contrast high scores on rational culture generally showed *positive* (but weaker) correlations with largely the same sets of variables. Thus clan culture and rational culture appear to work in opposite directions on many variables, with clan culture displaying more and stronger associations in general than the other culture variables.

Overall (see summary in Table 5.9 (p. 173)) group/clan cultures were associated with fewer complaints and better staff morale, and seemed to be present in smaller trusts characterized by lower amounts of activity, shorter waiting lists and less involvement in teaching and research. In general, the reverse was true for rational cultures. These findings fit with the competing values model as laid out in Boxes 5.1 and 5.2, where clan and rational cultures are diametrically opposed. Thus we would expect clan cultures to be more internally focused on maintaining group cohesion (e.g. morale) and this is likely to be easier in smaller institutions that can maintain a certain insularity (focused on local service delivery rather than engaged with the wider activities of teaching and research). In contrast, rational cultures adopt a more mechanistic approach to getting things done and are more competitive and outward looking.

The one further correlation of note is that staff satisfaction was moderately negatively correlated with hierarchical cultures (−0.33). Again, given the emphasis on rules, conformity and mechanistic processes in hierarchical cultures, and the clash of this with ingrained professional values around autonomy, such a finding helps confirm the plausibility of the competing values approach.

Model 3: ANOVA modelling of dominant culture and other trust variables

Many of the findings from the simple correlation analysis were confirmed by analysis of variance (for details see Model 3, Appendix 2). The one-way ANOVA approach used rational culture as the reference category and then 'least squares' to fit a linear model based on the unweighted data (the weighted model was also run but as this did not change the results significantly the data are not included).

Again, most statistically significant findings related to clan cultures and were entirely consistent with the correlation analysis (see summary in Table 5.9). In addition, these data suggested that waiting times were shorter in hierarchical cultures – perhaps consistent with hierarchical values of order, conformity and predictability.

Overall, the descriptive analysis provides good evidence for the face and construct validity of the competing values framework. Culture *did* vary across trusts using this measure, and at least some of this variation was associated in consistent and predictable ways with a variety of trust characteristics, including some performance measures (e.g. fewer complaints and better staff morale in clan cultures). We now move on to explore more closely relationships of culture with performance. Those variables that had higher correlations with various culture scores, and those that appeared as significant in the ANOVA results (largely the same), together with any *a priori* testable hypotheses (as set out in Table 5.1) were used to inform these later models.

Model 4: Explaining culture type by trust characteristics (multi-nomial logit modelling)

In Model 4 we explain differences in culture type using a number of the trust variables identified during the descriptive analysis and *a priori* hypothesizing. We were not able to combine the separate culture scores for each trust into a single dependent variable for the model and therefore used the dominant culture type in the first instance as the dependent variable. (This amounts to a loss of information since trusts proportionally may belong to one culture type more than another, but not exclusively to one. Econometrically we

Table 5.9 Trust characteristics associated with clan cultures (negative relationships) and rational cultures (positive relationships)

Area	Measures associated	Comments
Outcomes	• Complaints • Staff opinions	*Fewer complaints and better staff satisfaction in clan trusts compared to rational.*
Process measures	• Activity, such as: total spells, episodes, inpatient days, numbers of electives, emergencies, A&E attendances, first outpatient attendances, etc. • Waiting list variables (such as total inpatients waiting, and those waiting 3 and 6 months)	*Less activity and shorter waiting lists in clan cultures.*
Trust structural characteristics	• Size variables (such as bed numbers, free beds, sites with more than 50 beds) • Staffing variables (such as WTE doctors and other staff) • Expenditure variables (such as total cost, non-salary expenditure, total NHS, overall salaries)	*Trusts with dominant clan cultures were generally smaller and less involved in teaching and research; also they were less likely to have been merged.*

do not have a satisfactory way of dealing with this in a single model, since the culture scores are essentially jointly determined and constrained dependent variables.)

Modelling nominal outcomes in this way employs a multi-nomial logit approach (see details of Model 4, Appendix 2). Star ratings for zero and one star trusts combined were used as these provided the best results (since zero star trusts had small numbers), while two and three star categories remained insignificant in all specifications. Using bed numbers controlled for size and proved significant in all specifications, hence salary expenditure variables were adjusted to reflect relative proportions of total salary expenditure (so as not to also pick up size effects).

The findings demonstrate a number of significant relationships between culture, trust characteristics and trust performance. For example, clan culture trusts are less likely to have merged, are smaller (e.g. bed size) and tend to spend less on consultants and more on nurses. Perhaps unsurprisingly, management salaries were seen to be highest in those trusts that were identified as hierarchical. Beyond these structural relationships, the results also provide important evidence that performance (broadly defined) may vary in contingent ways between trusts with different dominant cultures. For example:

- Zero and one star ratings were more likely in trusts with clan and rational cultures than in those with developmental cultures.
- Inpatient surveys on dignity and respect yielded higher scores in trusts with clan cultures than in trusts where the other three cultures were dominant.
- Staff opinion (morale) was higher in clan culture trusts than in rational culture trusts.
- Waiting times were higher in trusts with clan, developmental and rational cultures compared to hierarchical cultures.
- Research activity was higher in trusts with developmental, hierarchical and rational cultures compared to those with clan cultures.
- The level of specialization was higher in trusts with clan and rational cultures compared to developmental and hierarchical cultures.
- Data quality appeared to be better in clan, developmental and rational culture trusts compared to hierarchical trusts.

Other variables that were significant in the ANOVA results and correlations, or suggested from the testable hypotheses, were not significant in the multi-nomial logit. These include complaints, staffing numbers, activity, teaching status, casemix, information governance, trust in staff and financial balance. The weighting variable (number of respondents) was also tested as a potential explanatory variable, since the number of respondents in a trust may be associated with the culture in terms of people being more enthusiastic or responsive to outside requests. This variable was also, however, insignificant.

Model 5: An ordered probit model linking trust culture and trust star ratings

Star rating are the most general overall performance rating used for NHS acute trusts, a headline measure that has wide implications for that institution's future management and accountability arrangements, as well as its reputation. We were concerned therefore to assess further the relationship between senior management team culture and trust star ratings.

To test the relationship between trust cultures and trust star ratings we used an ordered probit model (for details see Model 5, Appendix 2). Since most of the process and outcome variables were in fact used to construct the star ratings, the only variables included in the model are structural variables, which for the most part can be considered exogenous in the shortrun. As expected, most of the structural measures included in the model are not significant in explaining any of the variation in star ratings, but it could be argued that these factors should be controlled for, nonetheless, to assess the 'pure' effect of culture on performance. In this model the culture scores are used (as opposed to culture type) in order to use the most available information on culture.

The results seem to be consistent with the multi-nomial logit results presented previously and suggest that higher star ratings (two or three stars) are less likely in trusts with clan, hierarchical and rational cultures than they are in trusts with developmental cultures.

CONCLUDING REMARKS

We began this chapter by posing three questions. First, *can senior management team culture in the NHS acute sector be assessed?* Second, *is senior management team culture related to organizational characteristics and performance?* And third, *is there evidence that any such relationships are contingent?* The answer to all three of these questions would seem to be, *yes.* Thus these data provide significant extensions to the evidence-base linking culture to performance in health care (Chapter 2) as well as extending the generalizability of the findings derived from the case studies (Chapters 3 and 4).

Overall, the descriptive analysis provided more evidence for the face and construct validity of the competing values framework. Culture *did* vary across trusts using measures derived from the CVF, and at least some of this variation *was* associated in consistent and predictable ways with a variety of trust characteristics (e.g. size and merger status) and performance (e.g. complaints, staff morale, waiting times and even star status). Furthermore, clan culture dominance and rational culture dominance were associated with largely the same set of variables, but in reverse directions, which was again consistent with the underlying structure of the CVF.

In terms of these results confirming or refuting *a priori* hypotheses, the findings seem to be plausible. They provide particular support for a contingent relationship between culture and performance. For example, we might expect organizations with dominant clan cultures to be more internally focused and hence potentially poorer performers on formal external measures of success. This was borne out in the study: these organizations were smaller, more resistant to mergers, had a higher degree of specialization and were more concerned with staff morale and with treating patients with dignity and respect. Dominant developmental culture seemed to be associated with proportionally higher consultant and nurse salaries, which may relate to greater concern for clinical innovation and entrepreneurship and clinical teams being given greater freedoms and responsibilities. Hierarchical cultures seemed to be associated with proportionally higher management salaries, which may reflect the greater emphasis on the role of managers in establishing rules and procedures. Two contradictory findings here are that a hierarchical culture was associated with poorer and not better data quality, which may relate to the flow of information being poorer in this type of trust. We also note lower waiting times in these trusts, which we may have instead anticipated more with the developmental culture (perhaps being more innovative with the clinical management of waiting lists). Thus it may be the case that rules and procedures are a better way to manage waiting lists than innovation and entrepreneurship (it should however be recognized that management of waiting times will extend far beyond what we can observe from these four organizational culture typologies). Finally, as expected, the dominant rational culture trusts were more externally focused, bigger, less concerned with staff morale and more interested in research activity.

Different dominant senior management team cultures also seemed differently able to deliver on the broader assessments of performance embodied in star ratings, with dominant developmental cultures being more likely to deliver two or three star ratings. Thus we found significant relationships between culture and performance even using blunt 'bundled' measures of performance (the star ratings) and simple measures of culture (20 questions asked of a handful of senior managers in each trust).

Taken together then, these findings display a remarkable degree of consistency with the hypothesis that organizational culture is related to performance in a contingent manner – i.e. that those aspects of performance valued within the dominant culture are those aspects on which the organization will excel. They therefore reinforce findings from important previous work carried out across the USA, the UK and Canada (Gerowitz *et al.* 1996), as well as confirming the wider applicability of the case study findings previously presented. Both *a priori* hypothesizing and *post hoc* reasoning (based on an understanding of the values underlying various culture types) demonstrate relationships in hypothesized or plausible directions. That these relationships are found when culture is assessed simply using the perceptions of a small cadre of senior managers is indicative of both the central importance of senior management in trusts and the power of culture. Moreover, the relationship of culture with star ratings – suggesting that trusts with a dominant development culture are better able to achieve high star status – is even more remarkable, and certain to be of interest to both policy makers and change agencies.

Of course, interpretation of these findings should be tempered by a degree of caution. First, and most obviously, we only assessed culture by exploring the views of senior managers. Whilst we would in no way suggest that such an approach can capture all important cultural aspects of organizations, we believe it to be justified given the agenda setting powers and influence of the senior management team. Of course, the focus that we have chosen does not obviate the need for deeper study that explores how the dynamics of culture are played out at other layers within the organization. Second, these findings emerge from cross-sectional work. This clearly limits presumptions of causality that would be better substantiated through longitudinal study. Moreover, even if culture and performance are seen to co-vary we have few grounds for presupposing any particular direction of causality: it seems equally plausible that certain cultures may emerge in high performing organizations as it does that extant culture will drive performance. More intriguingly still is the potential for culture and performance to exhibit recursive relationships. Such complex and bi-directional relationships are of course better investigated through multi-method approaches that draw to a large degree on qualitative methods (and indeed supportive findings in this respect are reported from the intensive case studies on selected sites).

Third, our measures of both culture and performance suffer from limitations and may be contested: significant further development in each of these areas would be valuable to underpin future research.

Despite such methodological reservations, these findings indicate that organizational culture may indeed matter in the delivery of high performance in health care; they even go some way towards suggesting which sorts of cultures might be expected to enhance which aspects of performance. The real challenge will lie in encouraging an appropriate *blend* of local cultures, a blend that best manages to balance the tensions between underlying cultural values, and thus enable delivery across a wide spectrum of performance. More likely is that this is not readily achievable, and trade-offs will have to be made. Thus, policy makers, senior managers and other important stakeholders might take the view that certain aspects of performance are those that should be most highly prized – and they may then seek to inculcate those cultural values that best promote these aspects of performance.

NOTE

1   The details of each model developed are included in Appendix 2. The main text focuses on drawing out the key findings and their interpretation.

6

FINDINGS FROM THE PRIMARY CARE CASE STUDIES

(with Liz Nelson)

INTRODUCTION

The preceding chapters have focused on explaining culture in acute hospital settings. However, we were also interested in extending these ideas to primary care settings. As a result we carried out additional fieldwork in six primary care trusts (PCTs). In this chapter we present insights derived from the six PCT case studies.

PCTs are very different organizations from the acute trusts described in Chapters 3, 4 and 5. They are newer, less well structured and, in terms of their core staff, smaller than acute trusts. In their role as purchasers of secondary care and both providers and purchasers of primary care services, PCTs serve a quite different function from the focused activity of hospitals on the provision of well-defined acute services. The political focus on primary care is also less sharp than that on secondary care, and there are far fewer official performance data available. As a result, relatively speaking at least, PCTs are not at present under the same degree of pressure to be seen to 'deliver' on political imperatives.

It would therefore not have been appropriate for us to use the same case study methods in the two sectors. The key methodological differences were the smaller number of interviews conducted in PCTs (reflecting the smaller management teams) and the move straight to an integrative analysis rather than the production of single organization case narratives. Further methodological details are given in Appendix 1. In addition to these differences in the nature of the organization, and therefore potentially the culture, we conducted the primary care case studies in the knowledge that the concept of 'performance' might be viewed quite differently by PCTs and acute trusts. We therefore start this chapter with a brief reflection on the background to and concept of the term 'performance' in primary care.

DEFINING 'PERFORMANCE' IN PRIMARY CARE ORGANIZATIONS (PCOs)

The lower profile of primary care and the lack of high quality performance indicators relevant to PCOs' main functions dictates that the concept of performance in PCTs is likely to be less explicit than that for acute trusts. Much of what primary care providers do has traditionally been dictated by the professionals themselves, and assessment of performance has often been largely implicit. However, as performance management becomes more prevalent in the NHS, this is starting to change. The following section describes what changes have been implemented so far, and what is on the horizon.

In February 2002 the Department of Health published a new set of performance indicators for health authorities. Many of these had a population, and some a primary care, focus. However, the majority were dependent on secondary care data such as admission and referral rates. With the demise of the health authorities and the recognition of the increasingly important role played by PCTs, these indicators were adapted and relaunched for PCOs in September 2002 (see Box 6.1). Data relating to the performance of these PCOs were published on the Department of Health website (www.doh.gov.uk/ performanceratings2002) – though star ratings were not developed at this stage because of the perceived problems of attribution to such new organizations.

Since April 2003 responsibility for devising and publishing performance ratings has passed to the Office for Healthcare Information, part of the Commission for Health Improvement which was responsible for producing the first set of PCT star ratings in the summer of 2003. The Office becomes part of the new regulatory agency, the Commission for Healthcare Audit and Inspection in April 2004. The Department of Health continues to have an input into the indicators chosen. Attempts are currently being made to develop a set of indicators more relevant to primary care, more attributable to PCOs and more balanced towards outcomes. However data problems, in terms of both accessibility and quality, continue to inhibit attempts to produce a meaningful set of primary care

---

Box 6.1 PCO performance indicators for 2001/2002

Access to quality services
- Number of patients waiting over 15 and 18 months for inpatient treatment
- Number of patients waiting over 26 weeks for an outpatient appointment
- Surgery to remove cataracts
- Surgery for coronary heart disease
- Surgery to replace joints, including hips and knees

Service provision
- Percentage of patients able to see GP within 48 hours
- Patients' satisfaction with services available from GP, as measured by survey
- Number of GPs who have access to Internet
- Deaths caused by accidents
- Emergency admissions for those suffering from, e.g., asthma or diabetes
- Prescribing levels of generic drugs
- Prescribing levels of antibacterial drugs
- Prescribing levels of ulcer healing drugs

Improving health
- Deaths from circulatory disease
- People who have quit smoking after 4 weeks
- Levels of sexual health as measured by numbers of diagnoses of gonorrhoea
- Teenage pregnancy measured as conceptions under the age of 18
- People screened for cervical cancer
- Children immunized against measles, mumps, rubella and diptheria
- People vaccinated against flu

---

indicators. This problem will be partially addressed when data arising from the implementation of the new GP contract becomes available.

The extent to which the PCOs themselves engage with this explicit performance agenda has not hitherto been formally investigated. Given the aims of this project – to examine the relationship between organizational culture and performance – this issue was therefore addressed explicitly in the PCT case studies.

OVERVIEW OF KEY THEMES

We identified seven key themes from the case study data relating to the aims of the study:

1 managerial perceptions of cultural change and performance in PCTs;
2 the cultural characteristics of general practice;
3 improving the performance of PCTs by encouraging collaboration and partnership between practices;
4 improving the performance of PCTs by developing external partnerships;
5 improving the performance of PCTs by working with the public and with patients;
6 the use of different strategies to change performance;
7 constraints or obstacles to cultural change.

The rest of this chapter describes and interprets these themes.

Managerial perceptions of cultural change and performance in PCTs

Managers described PCTs as organizations that were trying to find new meanings for themselves. This term reflected their desire to distance themselves from what they perceived to be the old paternalistic and bureaucratic culture of the NHS and develop what they described as a new corporate identity.

> We've inherited a bit of culture from the Health Authority, the Community Trust and from primary care. What we are trying to do in developing a new culture is to take the best and leave the worst of those aspects and to try to bring them together to create a corporate identity for the organization.
>
> (Chief executive)

> We've gone from many islands in our archipelago to a feeling that we've got less completely off-shore interests and more of a [need for] confederation-building.
>
> (Chief executive)

The corporacy of this new organization was manifest by the desire for greater sharing of ideas, resources and data between practices. The new meanings reflected a perceived need for greater openness and transparency, a desire to focus on continuous learning, and a wish to create an environment in which mistakes were used as opportunities for learning, rather than opportunities to apportion blame.

> It's more a case of thinking as an organization as a whole, being prepared to do things together, being prepared to learn together, share things, all of which didn't exist before – of wanting to do things together and being more comfortable doing it.
>
> (Clinical governance lead)

> The culture I want to promote is to challenge and to put ourselves under the spotlight when acknowledging our weaknesses but congratulating ourselves when we've done well. That sort of culture is going to be so important and it fits with modernizing the service – challenging the way we provide patient care – and it will be good for all of us.
>
> (Director of LHG)

The managers spoke principally about the need for these new values to be manifest by general practitioners and their staff. Few of the interviewees suggested that there might be a need for their own management culture to change as well.

The majority of PCT managers do not view the term 'performance' in the same way as the acute trust managers. They perceived that the emphasis on the performance of their organizations at such an early developmental stage should be judged by their ability to build strong relationships and to facilitate cultural change. They thought that this was more important than their performance with respect to specific issues such as those in the National Performance Assessment Framework or a system of star ratings. This confirms the findings of an earlier study in the same PCTs (Marshall *et al.* 2002).

Most of the managers regarded changing culture as *the* key performance issue as far as they were concerned. So, unlike the acute trust managers, they made very few references in the interviews to the performance targets currently being used by the Department of Health. Several interviewees stated explicitly that they were using objective tasks, such as implementing the National Service Frameworks, principally as vehicles for changing culture. The managers recognized the resulting tension between what they regarded as 'real change on the ground' and the demands for measurable change being made by the Department of Health. Several of them described their roles as 'buffers' between the Department of Health and the practices in order to deal with this tension. They suggested that improved performance using objective measures would follow on from cultural change and would only be achieved and sustained if that cultural change was achieved.

Most participants thought that the development of a corporate culture amongst GPs would require significant compromises from both the GPs and the managers and would not be achieved quickly:

> This is the most fundamental change that has taken place since 1948 when the NHS first came into being. So not surprisingly it will take time, and if you have grown up in a culture of fierce independence it's very difficult to suddenly become a corporate being, so you have to convince GPs of the benefits of joining the club.
>
> (Chief executive)

Three of the PCTs in the study were formed by merging smaller PCGs. Several participants commented on the different cultures of these earlier organizations and the challenges of working across these cultures. Some had addressed the problem by formally establishing locality groups, with boundaries similar to the previous PCGs, and actively encouraging different approaches from these groups:

> Organizational culture is important and it exists but it isn't homogeneous in this organization. The three localities have got different cultures and we've deliberately given them autonomy so they can have their own culture if they want it. We have some over-riding principles that we would like to instil, but that's as far as it goes.
>
> (Chief executive)

The cultural characteristics of general practice

The managers readily identified what they perceived to be the cultural characteristics of the practices within their PCTs (Box 6.2). These values are characteristic of the clan-type culture in the competing values framework (Cameron and Freeman 1991; see Chapter 5, p. 161). In particular the cultural characteristics predominantly reflect those of inward looking organizations which are resistant to change. This has significant implications for the modernization agenda which requires a dynamic primary care sector to drive change across the whole health system. Some of the participants referred to the benefits of the cultural characteristics to patients and to the NHS, though others spoke about the negative impact of the values on the managers' ability to improve the performance of their PCT.

Box 6.2   Managers' perceptions of the current cultural characteristics of general practice

A sense of history and tradition: manifest by an awareness of the work that has gone into building a practice and a feeling that 'we've always done things this way and don't see any reason to change for change's sake'. A feeling that new initiatives come and go but that general practice goes on unchanged.

A sense of cohesiveness and loyalty to the practice as an organization: manifest by a tendency to support the practice in preference to any other organization.

A strong orientation towards professional autonomy: manifest by a suspicion of anything that potentially erodes this autonomy.

A tendency to be inward-looking: manifest by a resistance to work with, compare or learn from, other practices.

A tendency towards paternalistic leadership styles: manifest by a lack of strong and radical leadership at a practice level.

Improving performance through collaboration and partnership between practices

Given the broad definition of performance used by the PCT managers, the interviewees tended to focus their contribution on their strategies for improving collaboration between practices. Most managers were generally positive about the progress that they were making in getting practices working together on clinical governance issues. However, they were frustrated that whilst they were able to engage GPs over clinical matters relating directly to individual patients, they found it far more difficult to engage them with the PCT's agenda relating to a more proactive, population-based approach to delivering care. They explained these problems in terms of the nature of the training and the motivation of doctors choosing general practice as a career and felt that this was a significant barrier to improving the health of the local population. In addition, many thought that there was still considerable resistance to cross-practice working amongst a large number of general practitioners.

Some of the interviewees, particularly the middle managers, tended to address this lack of engagement by adopting a sympathetic, mentoring, facilitating style of working. They tended not to challenge established cultural norms, even when they believed them to be inappropriate:

> We have one practice which has all along believed that clinical
> governance was rubbish . . . I have never challenged them and
> never had an argument with them that their view of the world is
> not right because I think that if we can get them by action to
> change . . . they will realize that they have changed without me
> having to rub it in.
>
> (Clinical governance lead)

Middle managers believed that this approach offered the greatest
chance of overcoming GP resentment at being 'managed' and being
'forced' to work with other practices. At the same time, they recognized that such an approach took time and was unlikely to engage
those practices that were particularly resistant to change. These
managers expressed a particular dilemma in their dealings with practices that they considered to be providing a good quality service to
their patients, but which refused to engage with the corporate PCT
agenda. There were several of these practices in most of the study
sites and the managers found them particularly frustrating because
of the missed opportunities for less well performing practices to
learn from their expertise.

In contrast to the approach adopted by the majority of middle
managers, there were indications that most senior managers were
more in favour of authoritative working styles in their attempts to
achieve greater uniformity between practices. One chief executive
spoke of his willingness to challenge what he regarded as rigid,
inappropriate cultural traits, such as the desire of GPs to remain
autonomous. Whether this was the result of senior managers' roles
as agents of the Department of Health, or whether it reflected their
personal preferences, is unclear from this study. This issue is
addressed in more detail below.

Improving the performance of PCTs by developing external partnerships

PCTs have a wide range of responsibilities, including developing
partnerships with other organizations in the health and non-health
sectors. Again, the development of these partnerships was seen as an
important part of any judgement of their performance as an organization. Most of the discussion about such partnerships focused on
relationships with Departments of Social Services and other agencies within local authorities. PCT managers recognized the policy
priority of developing new partnerships and the inherent difficulties

of doing so. They felt that alliances should be forged first at a senior and strategic management level, rather than at the level of individual general practices:

> I think those relationships are having big enough problems being developed at the macro-organizational level, that is with the PCTs, the Council and Social Services and so on. I think it's quite unrealistic to expect local practices to develop these sorts of links. The practices use those services but they are there as services which they tap into and use when they need to. I think at the moment the way forward is to encourage and make links with outside agencies at the higher level first and when that's successful I think it might spread down.
>
> (Chair of LHG)

One of the main barriers to working with local authorities was felt to be the different cultures of the two organizations. One of the PCTs was attempting to address this problem by seconding staff:

> Councillors are so autocratic, their culture is so different from ours . . . The process in the council is so different to the process in the health service . . . We're going to have a councillor seconded onto our board, probably one of the non-execs will go onto one of their area committees, so we develop together – it's about developing trust.
>
> (Non-executive lead)

Structural barriers were also considered to be a major problem, particularly the existence of separate budgets:

> There's great potential to share with Social Services and pool budgets. One of the areas we've done that is learning disability and that actually has a pooled budget now. Things like community equipment for example would work well with a pooled budget.
>
> (Director of nursing)

It was clear that some PCTs were considerably more advanced in their partnership development than others. One chief executive talked of the difficulty in achieving the right balance in investing time and resources into the development of 'joined up partnerships' without losing sight of the PCTs' role in supporting primary care.

A second area of interest in external collaboration for the PCTs concerned the development of partnerships with other PCTs. There was a feeling that PCTs tended to work in isolation and missed opportunities to support each other and learn from each other's experience. One PCT chair spoke of an initiative to establish a 'think tank' with other PCTs for the purpose of sharing, learning and lobbying for recognition:

> We have a learning set of four PCTs, we meet in London, pick up various topics, no minutes, all completely confidential and it's brilliant. The chairs have become a sort of lobby group – and because there are four of us together – it develops credibility, a sort of gravitas that you don't have to churn on your own. Last time we got churned up about training, about the quality of it, so I was chosen to write off to the Commission and they take us seriously.
>
> (PCT chair)

Improving the performance of PCTs by working with the public and with patients

Since the development of relationships was considered to be a key facet of the performance of PCTs, we explored this issue with respect to public involvement. Whilst greater patient involvement in the NHS is an important policy imperative and regarded by the Department of Health as a key area of performance for PCTs, it was not one of the major themes emerging from this study. The few references that were made to it suggested that they were experiencing significant problems and that little progress was being made. One manager felt that her PCT was wasting time and money trying to fit in with government policy in this area. The lay member of the PCT board is expected to take a lead role but this did not seem to be happening. Particular concerns were expressed about the extent to which current PCT lay members were really able to represent the public:

> I don't believe our lay representatives are our real patients. Somebody gave me the view that most of our patients – the ones who really need care and treatment – are the ones with dirt under their fingernails and a drug problem and are beaten up regularly and their husbands are in prison. These are really difficult patients to engage and unless we are finding ways to commission their peers to represent them, we're not going to get a proper view, because our views are biased by our backgrounds.
>
> (Director of LHG)

We have at least one lay member of the population on our clinical governance board. Now it's a criticism that these are not necessarily representative members of the population but you have to strike a balance between Joe Public and someone able to understand the issues and able to be comfortable with the group. They must feel they are sitting amongst peers and be able to challenge us effectively.

(Clinical governance lead)

It appears therefore that the concept of developing relationships as a performance issue for PCTs focuses principally on practices, then on external agencies and other PCTs, and last of all on partnership with the general public.

The use of different strategies to change performance

In terms of their approach to addressing performance issues, it would be an over-simplification to suggest that there is a homogenous 'management perspective' within PCTs. Tensions between different managers, and in particular different layers of management, were evident. Notable disagreements were found in five of the six study sites. These differences of opinion were less likely to be recognized and voiced by the senior managers (the executive directors) than by the middle managers (all other managers, including the clinical governance leads).

The differences can be explained principally in terms of communication problems and preferred working styles of middle and senior managers. Middle managers described themselves as the 'workers' and felt that they were excluded from the strategic thinking of senior managers. Communication problems were exacerbated in two of the sites by geographical problems because the senior managers and middle managers worked from different buildings:

The difficulty we suffer from in this PCT is the fact that half the management – who are the most senior people – are housed elsewhere and the other [management] people who are doing all the work, are here. This is completely ridiculous. The executives don't want to come in this building because it was the old community trust building, but they've cut their nose off to spite their face because if they were upstairs – where there is a whole floor – communication would be better.

(Clinical governance co-ordinator)

The tensions were particularly notable in the PCTs that had recently undergone mergers:

> I think middle managers always feel a little vulnerable in any re-organization. It's not anybody's fault but it's taken a while for the executive directors to be put in post and we haven't got a structure yet so they feel displaced and not sure where they fit in the organization. I think the other issue is about the culture of the organization and middle managers not feeling belonging and feeling that they are not being communicated with – communication is an issue.
>
> (Director of service modernization)

There was evidence that some senior managers were sensitive to these tensions:

> I think the middle managers are more important because they represent the PCT and they're the first line of contact and if you look at all the organizational theory and if you look at those organizations who do really well, they invest in their middle managers and we've not done that. It's been very typical of an NHS organization – it's very hierarchical and almost authoritarian from that perspective, so we've got to do something to address that.
>
> (Director of service modernization)

Iterative analysis of the interview transcripts suggests that most PCT managers want to develop a culture amongst their practices manifest by a willingness and ability to embrace change, demonstrate flexibility and take risks. These are the characteristics of the 'open' culture described by the competing values framework. This cultural destination contrasted with the 'clan' culture that they considered to be currently predominant in general practice. The term 'clan culture' describes the characteristics of loyalty, tradition and cohesiveness that are often found in professionally dominated organizations.

As described earlier in this section, the priority of one group of managers was towards relationship-building rather than achieving specific objective targets. This group of managers can be referred to as 'facilitative' managers and the style was particularly prominent amongst middle managers. The approach aligns closely with the soft systems methods used in networked organizations (Checkland 1994), where the process of encouraging dialogue between parties operates alongside, and sometimes takes precedence over, the achievement of specific tasks. This contrasts with the performance management approach characteristic of hierarchical organizations, where the use of rules, policies and targets predominate. The culture survey demonstrated that a hierarchical culture is weak in general practice, particularly from the viewpoint of the general practitioners. Using approaches aligned to this cultural type is therefore likely to lead to conflict.

The approach adopted by the facilitative managers suggests that they prefer to work with the prevailing clan culture of general practice in order to meet the government objectives, rather than to directly challenge it. This could represent an unwillingness to challenge vested interests, or it could be explained in terms of a perception of the most effective way of achieving change in the context of general practice.

Facilitative managers are using a number of different strategies to stimulate culture change, which are aligned to their philosophical approach. For example considerable emphasis was placed on the value of them visiting practices in person:

> The locality manager, the director and myself go round and visit each practice and we discuss what problems they might have. Before decisions are made, we consult with practices about how they feel. It's a bit time consuming but it's worthwhile because at the end of the day, the value of any relationship or the way it develops is based on the amount of communication between parties. If managers are just stuck away in offices dictating from the centre, then clearly you are not going to have the same collaboration or co-operation as you would have if people meet and discuss problems on a regular basis.
>
> (Chair of LHG)

> If people distrust me and my motives then I am not going to get anywhere, and if I give them any reason to distrust me then I've totally lost the cause. My motives are quite transparent – if I have concerns about a practice because of a certain issue within that practice I try to be as honest as I can be with the practice. It's a case of building up mutual trust and respect.
>
> (Director, locality group)

In addition, facilitative managers tended to make use of peers to encourage change. For example some spoke of asking respected opinion-leading GPs to visit practices and discuss their problems with clinical governance:

> We also bring outside GPs along so that our GPs don't think we are trying to put one over on them! We bring GPs from other

areas who have had successes with PMS and they are more ready to listen to GPs than they are to managers.

(Chief executive)

Another way to get them to share is where there is a GP that they respect, so we've got a GP in the city who is a bit of an expert on CHD among his peers – the Expert GP thing – and they will come out for him and listen and share with him because they see him as someone who knows what he's talking about.

(PCT chair)

Such an approach to achieving change is compatible with the social interaction theory described by Grol (1997). Facilitative managers also made considerable use of practice managers and practice nurses as conduits to the doctors. Practice managers were seen as having particular potential in this respect. Facilitative managers were encouraging practice managers to meet regularly, exchange ideas and contribute to PCT activities. In well-established practices the managers were regarded as the centre pin of the organization, having a key role to play in changing attitudes at a practice level and having 'a foot in both camps'.

I think there's a good deal of sharing at the practice manager level – it's about shared tips, about shared ways of doing things, it's about sharing best practice with each other – it's a big area and there's very little sharing between practices at doctor level. Practice managers are very keen and getting them to do things together can be a catalyst to getting GPs doing things together, or community nurses doing things together.

(PCT chair)

However, some GPs refused to allow their managers to make a significant contribution at PCT level:

It depends on the practitioners themselves and how much responsibility and how much freedom the practice manager has. There are still a couple here where the manager is not easily allowed to go out to meetings or other events because they should be working – because obviously they are being paid and employed by the doctors themselves and they consider their time should be spent in the practice.

(Clinical governance lead)

I think some practice managers can block or be resistant to change because they are squeezed between the GPs who are ultimately their paymasters and the PCT who seemingly applies top-down pressure and some of them perhaps have been put into positions where it's impossible to deliver.

(Locality manager)

Practice nurses were also seen as being more willing to share ideas between practices than their employing GPs. Facilitative managers were actively promoting this willingness, particularly in chronic disease management:

We've done a lot of work around CHD registers and primary collaboration and so on – and the original work – creating a lot more sharing amongst GPs about CHD – getting enthusiasm going – came from the nurses not from the GPs.

(Chair of PCT)

In contrast to this facilitative approach to managing change, another group of managers were more inclined to set specific targets and to attempt to achieve them using incentives and encouraging competition between practices. This group of managers can be referred to as directive managers and the style was particularly dominant amongst senior managers. It appears that whilst both facilitative and directive managers pay lip service to developing an open culture, the methods used by directive managers were incompatible with that cultural destination and were actually more aligned to operating within a hierarchical or rational culture (Cameron and Freeman 1991). Mixed messages are therefore being delivered by different PCT managers to their practices and this might be one of the explanations for the lack of cohesiveness between the PCTs and their constituent practices.

The differences in the approaches of facilitative and directive managers are summarized in Table 6.1.

Constraints or obstacles to cultural change

This chapter has highlighted a number of significant barriers to changing the traditional culture of general practices to the new open and collaborative culture that PCT managers think is most conducive to high quality performance in general practice. This final part summarizes these barriers using a framework described by Grol (1997). He classifies barriers to change into three categories: barriers relating to the individuals concerned, barriers relating to social factors and barriers relating to organizational factors. Whilst this

Table 6.1   Characteristics of directive and facilitative managers

	Directive managers	Facilitative managers
Approach	Revolution, challenge established values	Evolution, work with established values
Focus	Performance targets	Gaining trust, building relationships
Incentives	External, especially financial	Internal, especially protected time
Levers	Patients/public Executive position Political authority	Practice managers and practice nurses
Use of peers	Peer competition	Peer support
Perceptions of obstacles to cultural change	Individual blockers	Organizational or environmental impediments

taxonomy was designed to explain the resistance of individual clinicians to adopting new innovations, it can be adapted to categorize barriers to organizational cultural change. The main barriers are summarized in Box 6.3.

The PCT managers have been attempting to address the individual barriers to date, and have had some success in doing so. This chapter has described some of the strategies that they are using. Most of the constraints relating to the social environment, such as historical norms, are unlikely ever to be within the control of individual managers. There must be some doubt about the ability of any of them to be actively changed or manipulated, though some might change gradually over time. These barriers are probably the most important ones in terms of sustained change in the values that underpin organizational culture and its relationship to performance. Most of the organizational barriers to changing culture are also largely outside the control of local PCT managers and will therefore prove much more difficult to change without action taken higher up in the health service.

Box 6.3   Main constraints to cultural change (modified from Grol 1997)

Constraints relating to individuals:
- resistance of GPs to reduced professional autonomy (reflected in resistance to being 'managed' and to partnership working between practices);
- lack of specific skills and knowledge (for example in promoting greater user involvement).

Constraints relating to social environment:
- historical values and norms of NHS (for example professional dominance, secrecy);
- tensions between societal and professional/managerial expectations (for example patients' desire for continuity of care, but GPs' desire to reduce their working hours and managers' to introduce greater skill mix into frontline care provision);
- desire of GPs to balance professional and personal life (reduced out of hours commitments, recognition of impact of professional demands on personal health);
- patient demands incompatible with new NHS norms (for example demands for new technologies that lack clear evidence of cost-effectiveness).

Constraints relating to organizational factors:
- level of funding (particularly financial crises in PCTs);
- staff recruitment and retention problems (particularly doctors and nurses);
- re-organization/lack of stability (distracts attention away from cultural change);
- communication problems due to dispersal of staff on different sites.

CONCLUDING REMARKS

The most fundamental difference between the opinions of PCT managers described in this section and those of the acute trust managers described in earlier chapters is their definition of the term 'performance'. Acute trust managers focus on the performance criteria emphasized by the Department of Health, most of which are formal measurements and relate to specific processes or outcomes of the provision of care. In contrast, many PCT managers see these explicit measures as consequences of a deeper underlying process of cultural change within primary care. Some even went so far as to dismiss objective performance targets and to see their *raison d'être* as being agents for cultural change. This approach, reflective of 'soft systems management' (Checkland 1994), was particularly prominent amongst middle managers. In contrast with their senior colleagues, middle managers appeared to prefer to implement change by working with the prevailing clan culture of general practice, rather than challenging it or attempting to impose a new culture.

This stance on performance can be viewed from a number of perspectives. Some commentators might criticize the approach for lacking a sharp performance management edge, perhaps even reflecting a lower calibre of manager in primary care in comparison with their acute sector colleagues. Others might simply regard it as reflecting the lower profile of primary care in the NHS and claim that as political attention shifts to the provider function of PCTs, then managers will have to become more focused on measurable performance. Indeed, it is apparent that the introduction of the PCT star rating system after this fieldwork was conducted is indeed focusing PCT managers' attention on objective performance. Others still may see the stance as an enlightened one, a desire to lay a firm foundation for meaningful and enduring improvement in performance, rather than simply to implement 'quick fixes'. This study does not allow us to differentiate between these possible explanations but the issue certainly warrants further investigation.

7

SUMMARY, CONCLUSIONS AND IMPLICATIONS FOR POLICY AND RESEARCH

INTRODUCTION

In this book we have conceptualized health care organizations as organic social entities, infused with values and emerging from natural social processes. The metaphor of organizational culture focuses on that which is shared between people within organizations, for example:

- the beliefs, values, ideologies attitudes and norms of behaviour;
- the routines, traditions, customs, symbols, ceremonies and rewards;
- the meanings, narratives and sense-making.

These shared ways of thinking and behaving help define what is legitimate and acceptable within any given organization and guide the many discretionary behaviours of health care professionals.

Although the notion of organizational culture is now invoked frequently in the social science and popular management literature, it remains a contested concept, fraught with rival interpretations and eluding a consensual definition. This contestability, however, has not precluded culture change and management from becoming a familiar prescription in health system reform. Nowhere is this more apparent than in the UK health system where the centralized administration of the NHS has allowed opportunities for the national government to experiment with a top-down approach to instilling new values, beliefs and working assumptions in the organization. Thus, culture has been blamed for organizational-wide deficiencies in the NHS with 'cultural transformation' seen as one route (alongside structural and procedural change) to enhanced quality, safety and performance across the organization. However seeking performance improvement in the NHS through cultural renewal and regeneration assumes the following stepwise logic:

1 The NHS and its parts possess a discernible culture or cultures.
2 The nature of such culture(s) has some bearing on performance.
3 Such culture(s) are malleable and not impervious to change.
4 It is possible to identify cultural attributes that are facilitative of high performance (or at least pinpoint those which are damaging).
5 Policy makers and managers can design (an optimal mix of) strategies that influence the formation of beneficial culture(s).
6 The benefits that accrue from managed culture change will outweigh any dysfunctional consequences.

For the current thrust of government policy to be well founded therefore, each of these assumptions needs to hold. However, as was shown in Chapter 2, the empirical evidence to date to support this stepwise logic is flimsy at best.

REMINDER OF THE AMBITIONS OF THIS BOOK

This book reflects an ambition to strengthen the evidence base that underpins this topic. To that end we have explored the potential for purposive culture management by examining the relationship between organizational culture(s) and the performance of NHS trusts. Our primary aim has been to assess the extent to which the causal logic set out above is supported in the NHS. On the basis of the implicit causal assumptions we derived a number of key research objectives, which were addressed through empirical study, the findings of which are reported in Chapters 3 to 6:

• Identification and classification of organizational culture(s) within NHS trusts
• Examination of senior managers' vision(s) for culture change within NHS trusts, especially those changes linked to clinical governance
• Exploration of any empirical relationship(s) between the culture(s) of NHS trusts and their measured (and unmeasured) performance
• Identification of those aspects of culture that are amenable to meaningful managed change

- Identification of the levers and facilitators of culture change in health care organizations, and highlighting the key barriers and inhibitors to culture change
- Identification of any contextual factors (e.g. national health policies) that facilitate (or inhibit) the development of virtuous cultures in NHS trusts
- Assessment of any unintended and dysfunctional consequences of culture change programmes.

DRAWING TOGETHER THE EMPIRICAL WORK AND CONCLUSIONS FROM THE FINDINGS

We found overwhelming support across a broad range of stake-holders, both internal (e.g. managers and clinicians) and external (e.g. consumer advocacy groups, Royal College senior officers, union leaders), for utilizing ideas of culture change in reforming the NHS. Culture change was considered a crucial element in improving the working lives of staff, and in enhancing the quality and safety of care provided to patients and their carers. In addition, we documented many examples where culture change policies were believed to be having a positive impact on the organization (e.g. more openness, greater degree of patient-centred care, more team working and less restrictive practices). Thus there appears to exist a broad-based consensus on the direction of travel, whilst still being disagreement or difficulties around both the pace of change and the means of influencing that change. In addition, whilst ideas of culture change as a means of service improvement were widely supported, other aspects of the modernization agenda, such as the accountability framework and structural changes, were seen as potentially problematic for organizations aiming to change their culture.

In elaborating on these conclusions, we take in turn each of the key objectives listed above, collating and summarizing the findings from the various pieces of empirical work described in Chapters 3 to 6, which were in turn informed by the theory and literature reviewed in Chapters 1 and 2. The policy implications and research implications from these findings are drawn out subsequently.

The nature of culture in the NHS

Culture is complex, dynamic and contested. Whatever the approach that is taken in assessing culture, it can only ever give a partial glimpse of the 'value infused institutions' (Selznick 1957) that under-pin organizational life. The complex grouping, layering and subcul-turing that exist in organizations can never be fully captured. In this book we have focused largely on the culture of NHS managers, particularly senior managers. We took this focus, first, because limited resources precluded extending our view in any detail to wider service delivery groups and second, because an existing litera-ture suggests that senior managers are very important drivers of organizational cultures (Gerowitz et al. 1996; Gerowitz 1998; Davies et al. 2000).

The competing values framework (CVF) proved to be a useful tool for assessing the cultural landscape of NHS organizations. Using this instrument, we categorized around one-half of acute trusts (54 percent) as having a dominant clan culture at senior man-agement level, 30 percent as having a dominant rational culture, and relatively few as having either a developmental (11 percent) or a hierarchical (6 percent) dominant culture. In addition, all of the primary care practices studied evidenced a dominant clan culture. Using the in-depth case studies we dug deeper to uncover rich descriptions of organizational life at the heart of the NHS, in both primary and secondary care.

Visions for cultural change

Our Introduction outlined the visions for cultural change evident in current policy documents, as well as those emanating from the Kennedy Report: service cultures that are open, safe, patient-centred, team-based and accountable. These themes are clearly exer-cising senior management thinking in both acute and primary care settings. Drawing on the data from the acute trust and PCT case studies, managers articulated cultural aspirations around a number of key themes:

- The need for a stronger patient focus, shaping services around the needs of patients rather than the historical needs of service providers/health care professionals.
- A desire to create a stronger 'corporate' perspective amongst professional staff, with a consequent loosening of allegiances to external or parochial drivers. This is particularly the case in pri-mary care where PCT managers want practices to work more closely together, sharing experiences and information.

- The development of no blame cultures so that staff can feel safe and confident in reporting critical incidents and errors.
- Improved cultures of accountability and control in trying to get a grip on service delivery and meet the demanding externally driven performance agenda.
- Better transparency and openness, to allow a free flow of information, greater learning and better risk management.
- The creation of a dynamic 'can do' culture, by cultivating, rewarding and nurturing positive attitudes to innovation and performance improvement.
- Greater attention to the development of well functioning multi-professional teams.
- Devolution of autonomy once performance credentials have been attained as a means of freeing up local creativity and dynamism and overcoming the inherent limits of tight control.

The empirical relationship between culture and performance

Until now, evidence from the research literature for a link between organizational culture and organizational performance is surprisingly sparse. Reviews of the link in the commercial sector find little convincing evidence, and this is reflected also in previous studies of health care (of which there have been very few in the UK (see Chapter 2).

This book therefore provides important new evidence, finding as it does both significant quantitative associations between existing cultures and various aspects of measured performance (Chapter 5), as well as evidence of a variety of mechanisms whereby such associations may be mediated (Chapters 3 and 4). The CVF typology highlighted that different culture types may be more or less able to perform, depending on those aspects of performance that are valued within that culture. For example acute trusts with developmental cultures were less likely to be awarded poor star ratings; trusts with hierarchical cultures were more likely to perform well in terms of waiting times; and those with clan cultures scored better on measures of staff satisfaction. Whilst making inferences of causality from cross-sectional associations is highly problematic, the in-depth qualitative work provided good corroboration by highlighting many plausible mechanisms by which cultural expectations may influence patterns of working and hence performance. Moreover, the relationship of culture with star ratings – suggesting that clan and hierarchical cultures are less able to achieve high star status – is remarkable, and certain to be of interest to both policy makers and change agencies. We have also drawn attention to the ways in which performance and culture interact in an iterative manner, perhaps even being mutually constituted. For example highly visible performance assessments (such as star ratings) impacted on culture both directly (e.g. by influencing staff morale) and indirectly (through renewed management activity). *Thus while culture and performance do seem to be linked in important and substantive ways, such links are many, varied, contingent and bi-directional.*

In exploring aspects of performance, it further became clear that there is almost as much controversy about how to define perform-ance as there is about defining culture. In health care, performance remains difficult to measure and dependent on the purpose and per-spective of the evaluation. Serious anomalies can arise, adding to its contested nature; for example one of the acute case study trusts (D) was a low performer on the star ratings but scored very highly on the alternative (and itself controversial) Dr Foster ratings. Staff in the acute trusts frequently drew attention to such anomalies and expressed frustration at the blunt nature of such broad-based assessments as star ratings. In the PCTs, facilitating cultural change is seen as the key performance issue in itself; minimal attention was paid by PCT managers to the more objective performance issues that were the focus of acute trust managers. Thus elaborations of any culture/performance link demand more careful attention than has been given hitherto to the nature of the performance being assessed.

Aspects of culture amenable to managed change

Various aspects of trust culture appeared, from our case study work, to be amenable to purposive managed change. Progress was being made, to varied extents, in addressing each of the cultural aspects identified earlier under our heading 'Visions for cultural change' (see p. 200). Whilst direct action to change these cultural aspects were most often and most readily observed in the acute setting, senior managers in primary care were also working to engender change. Their main aims were to improve collaborations and part-nership working between practices within the PCT framework as one means of engendering a more consistent and effective corporate approach. However, whilst PCT managers think that they can create a conducive environment for cultural change, they do not think that they can actively manage that change. They hope, but are not certain, that real sustained cultural change will emerge from greater collaboration between practices.

LEVERS, FACILITATORS AND BARRIERS TO CULTURAL CHANGE

Acute trusts are utilizing a wide variety of strategies, tactics and specific initiatives to drive cultural change. These include training and educational initiatives, perhaps supported by external agencies such as the Clinical Governance Support Team or the Modernisation Agency. External assessments, such as star ratings and CHI inspections were being used as a means of galvanizing significant internal changes, more so when these were accompanied by senior management changes. Leadership, and especially a consistency between rhetoric and actions, was seen as influential in shifting embedded attitudes. This was exemplified by the new and supportive ways that critical incidents were being dealt with. Practical demonstrations of the value placed on health professional groups (particularly nurses and allied professional groups) were emphasized as one means of strengthening a safety culture. Attempts at change also went wider than the organization, with higher performers taking a very active role in the wider local health economy – nurturing partnerships with other local agencies to improve co-ordinated care. Thus culture change was being attempted through a wide variety of interlocking approaches, which in turn presented some of the greatest challenges, those of ensuring coherent and mutually reinforcing messages, and of avoiding potentially dysfunctional consequences (see pp. 86–8).

Primary care trusts were more focused in their attempts at managed culture change. Their main activities centred on promoting dialogue and encouraging 'relationship building' amongst the formerly distinct practices. They used a range of strategies, including arranging meetings between practices, practice visits and liaison with practice managers to achieve their aims. Thus managers were working with, rather than cutting across, the prevailing clan culture of general practice, seeking informal peer-to-peer contact as a means of achieving corporacy, rather than imposing performance measurement and management systems to drive change. PCT managers saw GP independent contractor status as a significant barrier to greater corporatization but also expressed concern about barriers to cultural change that they considered outside their control, particularly the amount and pace of structural reform in primary care.

Contextual factors and organizational cultures

The public context for health care performance has changed dramatically over the past decade. The rise of consumerism, a decline of deference in professional practice and the high profile of a range of medical scandals have brought health care performance and quality to the top of both public attention and the public policy agenda. Whilst managers in trusts recognized these shifts, and acknowledged the importance of delivering on the performance agenda, there was nonetheless considerable disquiet over the scale, frequency and rapidity of change. Thus the external context, most especially the whole performance and accountability framework driven from the Department of Health, was seen as both sometimes enabling and facilitating, and sometimes disabling, distracting and damaging (we discuss later the policy implications of this need to balance enabling and disabling facets of policy initiatives).

Unintended and dysfunctional consequences

As any management initiative may give rise to a range of unintended, unwanted and ultimately dysfunctional consequences, we sought evidence as to whether the current emphasis on culture change was producing such effects. Within the acute trusts there was significant evidence of damaging as well as beneficial change:

- *Tunnel vision*: focusing on measured areas sometimes distorted clinical priorities.
- *Bullying and intimidation*: the emphasis on performance and accountability was seen to create a demanding climate for staff which could sometimes extend into uncomfortable levels of pressure and coercion.
- *Loss of morale and erosion of public trust*: the publicity surrounding poor star status was thought to have had negative effects on trust staff and local user confidence.
- *Ghettoization or polarization*: some senior managers feared that good staff would be lost (or hard to recruit) to apparently poorly performing trusts, exacerbating potential performance differentials.

Whilst the evidence supporting the extent of these problems is at present sketchy, they nonetheless represent common concerns that, if substantiated, have serious policy implications for the national performance framework (see pp. 86–8). Even within primary care, where the level of measured scrutiny is significantly less, there were nonetheless some concerns about dysfunctional change. In particular, some managers questioned whether greater corporatization would result in less innovation from general practices.

In sum, the findings from the various empirical studies offer considerable support for the attention culture change is receiving in the policy arena. Whilst they may also have many implications for senior managers in various care settings we focus next on drawing out the key policy implications for the NHS.

Policy implications

This section draws on the preceding conclusions to identify and elaborate some of the key policy implications arising from the study findings.

Key finding 1: culture matters

Conceptualizing organizational life in terms of 'organizational culture' resonates with a wide variety of key stakeholders in health care and forms an intuitive way for them to understand their organizational dynamics. Thus the key overall finding from the empirical studies is that organizational culture matters, and is seen to matter, in the delivery of high levels of quality and performance in NHS acute trusts, and is likely to be of increasing importance in primary care trusts as they develop a stronger organizational focus. Managers at all levels, in both secondary and primary care, recognized the significance of culture and were either actively interested in shaping it or felt constrained by its pervasive influence.

Policy implication

There is some empirical justification to support the government's case for targeting culture change alongside structural and procedural reform to secure the desired improvements in health care performance.

Key finding 2: performance is an elusive concept

Current measures of health care organizational performance were seen as contestable at best. In particular, whole organization performance rating (such as the star system currently used for acute trusts) were seen as poor measures – neglecting as they do the potential for areas of excellence within overall low rated institutions, as well as pockets of failure hidden in high rated institutions. Thus, in application, when tied to sanctions, star ratings were seen as blunt tools with potentially bludgeoning effects. Indeed primary care managers go as far as to suggest that the actual management of cultural change should *itself* be judged as one aspect of their performance.

Policy implication

Policy makers should be very careful about how they report, interpret and act on performance information. Whilst good performance data can enable change, poor measures can easily be discredited. They may, for example, lead to unwarranted denigration or unjustified reassurance, provide perverse incentives, or lead to a wide range of dysfunctional consequences (see p. 213)

Key finding 3: organizational culture appears to be linked to performance in a contingent manner

Evidence from acute trusts suggests that those aspects of performance valued in the dominant culture are those aspects on which the organization will excel. Therefore, judgements over the virtuousness of cultural attributes are necessarily intimately connected to an identification of desirable organizational end points, which may differ between settings and change over time. Many of the organizational problems intrinsic to the NHS highlighted in this report may be attributed directly to 'cultural lag' – the misalignment between entrenched professional values and practices (that have been woven into the fabric of the organization and affirmed over decades) and the changing demands/expectations of both policy and the wider environment.

Policy implications

There is a need to develop appropriate cultures in health care organizations, cultures that are aligned with key policy objectives for the National Health Service. However, the evidence supporting a contingent relationship between cultures and performance suggests that trade-offs will have to be made between policy objectives, with cultures then shaped to fit the key priorities. As culture is so embedded in organizations, and is often slow to change, a degree of realism is needed about the extent to which cultures can be manipulated to align with fast changing policy. The identification of longer-term more enduring values may be more realistic.

Further, the appropriateness or otherwise of extant organizational health care cultures needs to be subject to regular review and assessment, and organizational cultures should be revitalized to reflect important emerging concerns and shifting priorities in the wider environment. Strategic drift may be addressed retrospectively (as with current efforts to transform and modernize the culture of the NHS) or prospectively (e.g. attempts to 'horizon scan' future changes in health care and wider society in order to predict the form that new cultural attributes should take), with an optimal mix likely to comprise a judicious mix of retrospective and prospective cultural alignment strategies. The scale of these tasks should not be under-estimated. There will also be a need to adopt an 'open systems' approach, where the NHS is recognized as interacting with, and growing organically alongside, the wider environment – rather than being seen as a hermetically sealed institution separate from its wider social, economic and political context. The Department of Health's Forward Strategy Unit would appear to be a useful organization for exploring these implications.

Key finding 4: there are important cultural differences between apparently high and apparently low performing NHS acute trusts

The cultural characteristics of acute trusts appear to be linked in a systematic way to their measured (and unmeasured) performance. Indeed, we were able to discern a clear patterning in the configuration of core cultural attributes across high and low performing trusts. Whilst assertions of causality would need to be tempered by a due appreciation of the methodological constraints, it is our contention that there is much to be learned from an examination of these patterns of divergence. The key points of departure may be grouped under five broad headings: leadership and management orientation, functionality of middle management, accountability and information systems, human resources policies, and relationships within the local health economy.

Policy implication

Each of these cultural factors needs to be addressed in any attempts to enhance the performance of acute trusts, and each are discussed in more detail below.

Key finding 5: leadership is paramount; requisite leadership style is a function of current performance

Leaders serve an important function in creating, embedding and transmitting desired cultural attributes (Schein 1985b). One of the most powerful mechanisms for communicating their beliefs and espoused values is what they themselves pay attention to, for example, what aspects of organizational activity they choose to involve themselves in, and in what and how they seek to measure, control, reward and sanction. The dominant style of senior leadership in acute trusts is likely to influence organizational performance profoundly. Moreover, desirable styles of leadership may depend crucially on the stage in the performance cycle the organization finds itself (in the same way that Churchill was considered a great leader in war but not as suitable for leading in the peace that followed).

Apparently high performing acute trusts were characterized by a tradition of strong, directive, top-down or transactional styles of management, where the emphasis has been on establishing robust systems for monitoring and improving organizational performance. Such trusts may decide that they wish to consolidate and build on their high performance position by gradually adopting more participatory and devolved styles of management. This is because there are limits to the performance improvements that can be wrung out of transactional systems and the only way to continuously improve would be to evolve towards more transformational approaches, which draw on intrinsic motivations and generate fewer transaction costs. The crucial factor here is that these organizations have the capacity, informational infrastructure and performance management architecture to facilitate devolution of power and responsibility away from the apex and towards frontline staff. To attempt to move towards more devolved and participatory styles of management in the absence of the above factors would likely result in serious dysfunctional consequences, as power would be devolved without sufficient lines of accountability and control to the centre.

In contrast, apparently low performing acute trusts were characterized by a lack of strong directive planning and lacked robust systems of information and performance management. These trusts are likely to require a strong dose of transactional management in order to turn around their performance. Only once robust systems have been in place and have had the opportunity of being continuously refined and adapted through use can the organization consider developing more participatory styles of management. To do so prematurely would risk courting serious dysfunctional consequences.

The concept of leadership in PCTs is more complicated than for acute trusts. A new style of leadership of networked organizations is almost certainly more likely to reap greater benefits than any attempt to introduce the styles seen in more conventionally structured organizations.

Policy implications

Attention should be focused on matching leadership styles to current performance needs. Those organizations with a history of meeting external targets, and having in place robust systems of performance management, may be in a position to develop more participatory styles of management where power and authority over operational matters are increasingly devolved from central control. In contrast, those organizations with a history of under-performance may require more focused transactional style leadership with an emphasis on introducing strong lines of upward accountability for performance. These ideas are congruent with the current policy emphasis on earned autonomy – however such ideas currently rest on the doubtful assumption that whole-organization performance can be reliably measured.

Finally on leadership, there was some evidence from our case studies of leaders 'taking their eye off the ball' within their trust, perhaps through being distracted by opportunities on a wider national stage. Thus the incentive context for trust leadership needs to be set so that senior managers are encouraged to give due attention to good stewardship (perhaps organized through the NHS Leadership Centre), with fewer distractions or opportunities for moving on and out as local problems begin to become apparent.

Key finding 6: a strong and empowered middle management tier seems to be an essential element of a high performing organization

Middle managers act as the ears and voice of senior managers who may, in their absence, become disconnected or remote from day-to-day operational matters. Middle managers act as buffers and interpreters between senior staff and frontline staff and are often more sensitive to the best way of producing real cultural change on the ground. They are the essential communicators of a performance focused corporate culture, as well as a means of embedding such a culture in daily activities. Their role is particularly important in those organizations that have not yet been able to inculcate 'can do' high performance values in frontline teams. Serious dysfunctional consequences may ensue in situations where middle managers are disempowered and have little input into senior decisions.

Policy implications

Attention should be focused on developing a well-resourced, empowered and effective cadre of middle management who can drive through change in organizations and feel able to challenge and question senior management decisions. Equally, as frontline teams become more performance focused and self-supporting, further attention should be given to ensuring that the middle manager's role can change from that of performance enforcer to performance coach and facilitator.

Key finding 7: high quality information systems underpin robust accountability systems

In the acute sector, high performing trusts have developed clearer lines of accountability for performance. Accountability in turn depends crucially on good information systems. In such trusts, senior managers have well developed areas of individual responsibility, and clear mechanisms for delivering on these. In contrast, trusts that are struggling to deliver on performance are characterized by underdeveloped information systems, diffuse lines of accountability and team-based (i.e. diluted) responsibilities.

Policy implication

There is a need to invest in effective information systems as a means of underpinning open, transparent and focused systems of accountability for performance. In particular, the quality of information flow in primary care is known to be poorer than that in the acute sector, and this in turn has implications for the style of accountability and control systems that can function in this environment.

Key finding 8: an active human resources function underpins the formation and maintenance of performance-conducive cultures

High performing acute trusts paid particular attention to the human resources function. In particular one of the more subtle, but potent, ways of communicating and nurturing desirable cultural traits amongst organizational members is the observed criteria by which organizations recruit, select, promote, retire or even ex-communicate staff. To improve their performance trusts may need to nurture a corporate perspective amongst professional staff, especially consultants, through training and development programmes.

Policy implications

The selection of staff to fit a performance culture needs developing and support. As the workforce supply is limited, such performance enhancing strategies may have limited application unless supported by wider initiatives to improve that supply and develop the existing workforce capacity.

Key finding 9: inter-relationships with the local health economy are important for securing high performance

The performance of acute trusts is highly inter-connected with the performance of the local health economy, which in turn may be influenced by the quality of inter-organizational relationships, co-operation and partnership working amongst local agencies. Those trusts that are well connected and proactive, particularly in terms of their relationships with their PCTs, are likely to reap benefits of improved performance around such important areas as waiting lists, re-admission rates and A&E performance.

Policy implication

Trans-organizational leadership is currently under-developed in the NHS. Policy makers need to develop incentives for senior managers for the adoption of a 'whole economy' perspective that promotes collaborative working. One way of addressing these concerns would be to incorporate some assessment of the quality of communications and interactions in the local health economy within current accountability arrangements. There is also a need to train and support key boundary spanners who work through networks and are given resources and freedoms to transcend traditional organizational boundaries.

Key finding 10: embedding desirable cultural traits in health care delivery organizations require an alignment of national and local policies

Although there were some differences in the fine details, external and internal stakeholders exhibited a remarkable degree of convergence over the desirable cultural traits that should be developed and embedded within health care delivery organizations. These centred on:

- promotion of a patient centred focus;
- improved transparency and openness;
- a 'no blame' non-punitive climate where staff feel safe to report errors;
- a concern for quality and safety;
- a corporate rather than a purely professional outlook; and
- team-based working.

All of the acute trusts in our case studies were actively seeking to engender these perceived virtuous cultural attributes amongst staff, and much national government policy was reported to be helpful in levering improvements within organizations. However we also found reports that national policy such as the 'naming and shaming' of under-performing trusts was inimical to the development of some desired attributes such as the creation of no blame cultures.

Policy implication

Central government policy should be better aligned with the concerns of delivery organizations to improve the quality, safety and performance of services provided to patients. One way of achieving this might be to consult more closely with heath care organizations (e.g. chief executives and wider) on the implications of national policies before these are rolled out nationally. This process already occurs to some extent, for example the chief executives of first-wave three star trusts are consulted by the Department of Health. However many of the worst problems are experienced by apparently low performance trusts and the consultation process should also be extended to these organizations.

Key finding 11: dysfunctional consequences of culture change are likely

The case studies identified a range of adverse side effects that had been induced by the government's programme of modernization and performance improvement. For example there were some concerns that low performing trusts were experiencing problems in retention and recruitment of key staff, and a belief that these problems were compounded by the negative publicity associated with a star rating system. There are concerns therefore that the star rating systems (and the introduction of foundation trusts) may lead to a two tier service and the ghettoization of organizations which would experience a spiral of decline as high quality staff would be attracted to (apparently) high performing trusts. We also heard reports of bullying, harassment and intimidation of staff to deliver the desired improvements in performance, a perceived decline in levels of public trust and the distortion of clinical priorities. These deleterious effects have the potential to undo or overshadow many of the positive aspects of culture change.

Policy implication

Dysfunctional consequences should be anticipated and closely monitored, with policies put in place that are designed to mitigate them. This should be undertaken in an open and transparent manner and, where problems are found, this needs to be clearly reported. Perhaps there is an independent role for CHAI in doing this.

---

*Key finding 12: surmounting the barriers to implementing successful
culture change requires co-ordinated policies targeted at both internal
and external influences*

The case studies highlighted a range of factors that were associated
with impeding or attenuating efforts at culture change. These
included the retention of 'old culture' staff in key positions, a lack of
resources to invest in change programmes, the influence of professional bodies such as the BMA and the Royal Colleges, and aspects
of wider government policy which were seen as not being conducive
to fostering beneficial change in health care delivery organizations. It
is clear that overcoming such hurdles will require a range of policies,
some internal and some external, to provider organizations. For
example changing the socialization processes associated with professional practice depends on national government intervention to
change long established training and education practice. In contrast
overcoming organizational inertia associated with dysfunctional
management may require more local interventions.

Policy implication

Securing alignment across the whole range of policy reform and
supporting initiatives is important if cultural change is not to be
attenuated, blocked or even negated.

DISCUSSION

This book has sought to sharpen thinking around the theory and
feasibility of planned culture change in health care. To that end we
have highlighted the contingent and dynamic nature of the relationships that exist between the culture(s) of NHS trusts and aspects of
their measured and unmeasured performance. Those looking for a
magic bullet or simple cultural prescription for the ills of the NHS
will therefore be disappointed: our study suggests that 'what works'
depends crucially on context, and on how and by whom efforts targeted at culture reform are evaluated and assessed. Thus a change in
context or evaluative position may well render a hitherto desirable
cultural attribute problematic or, at the extreme, dysfunctional.

Based on the evidence reported in this book we would counsel
against a 'one size fits all' approach to culture management in the

NHS and encourage the adoption of more nuanced strategies which seek to deploy a judicious mix of instruments and supporting tactics depending on setting and application. These can be divided into two broad policy dimensions, both internal and external to NHS organizations: styles of leadership and management practices within NHS organizations (see Table 7.1), and strategic approaches to performance management across the NHS (see Table 7.2). The intention is to obtain the best effects of all approaches whilst minimizing dysfunctional consequences. This means paying attention to contingencies, constantly adapting approaches as dysfunctional consequences start to outweigh the benefits, and living with paradox. Of course, this leaves muddle, confusion and contradiction as likely outcomes. We now pick out a few of the key issues identified in Tables 7.1 and 7.2 for further discussion.

Table 7.1   Leadership and management in NHS trusts

Area	*Seek mix and balance between*		*Comments*
Management style	Transactional management	Transformational management	The optimal style of leadership required in NHS is necessarily a function of context, current performance, purpose and level.
Management orientation	Corporate focus	Pro-professional	A corporate focus seeks better alignment of values and purpose across the organization. However excellence in practice is underpinned by professional values, which may in turn be undermined by loss of autonomy.
Middle management	Strengthen, empower	Slim down, remove	De-layering and removal of middle management 'bureaucracy' may leave important gaps and provide a limited managerial capacity to deliver performance improvements.

Table 7.2 Strategic performance management issues in the NHS

Area	Seek mix and balance between		Comments
Values	Retention (core values)	Renewal (new values)	It is important to recognize and celebrate existing values within the NHS that are conducive to high quality/good performance.
Accountability	Checking	Trusting	Excess scrutiny and monitoring imposes high transaction costs and may damage trust. However an excessive reliance on trust may lead to opportunism and corrupt behaviour.
Blame	Blame/ scapegoating	'No blame' culture	Although the shift towards no blame cultures is to be encouraged, blame (and thus the taking of responsibility) may sometimes be appropriate. The aim should be to foster just cultures where blame, if it is warranted, is handled fairly.
Performance data	Hard data	Soft intelligence	Hard data are rarely that hard and may (justifiably) be contested. Blunt tools can be expected to have blunt effects. In the clamour to develop external systems of checking verification and audit extreme care must be taken not to suppress, undermine or distort channels of 'soft' intelligence.
Performance perspective	Single organization	Whole health economy	If organizations stand or fall on their own performance then integrated working may be harder to achieve – yet a whole economy

Area	Seek mix and balance between		Comments
			perspective may weaken incentives and encourage free-riders.
Performance management	Vertical performance management	Horizontal management (across networks)	Current accountability frameworks emphasize vertical systems, whereas policy stipulations favour network-delivered care.
Targets for change	Externally driven	Internally generated	Local ownership of targets may be important in securing commitment.
Incentives	Sticks (sanctions)	Carrots (rewards)	Incentives matter, and need to be in alignment, yet they may not be the key drivers of professional practice.
Motivations	Extrinsic drivers	Intrinsic drivers	Too much focus on extrinsic drivers may crowd out intrinsic motivations; fewer external controls may enhance intrinsic motivations, but if these are not well aligned with those of the objectives of the centre they may lead to deleterious outcomes.
Resultant effects	Beneficial change	Dysfunctional effects	Unintended effects may dilute or negate beneficial changes. All culture change policies need be monitored not only in terms of the beneficial consequences they effect but also the unintended and dysfunctional consequences they inadvertently give rise to.
Driving forces	Centrifugal	Centripetal	Too little central direction may lead to drift; too much may stifle initiative.
Speed of change	First order change	Second order change	Change fatigue is an enduring concern.

Styles of leadership and management practices

Our findings suggest a strong relationship between trust leadership and trust performance. Furthermore it is evident that both trans-actional and transformational styles of leadership are important for beneficial organizational functioning. It would seem that the trick is to mix and match the appropriate style to the stage in the perform-ance cycle in which the organization finds itself. Thus our empirical evidence suggests strongly that transactional styles are most useful in situations where an under-performing organization requires strong central direction to establish a robust internal performance man-agement architecture. In contrast, high performing organizations with established performance management systems and a long his-tory of central direction and clear lines of accountability may bene-fit by developing more participatory and devolved leadership styles. Middle managers also play a crucial role in the levering performance improvements and, depending on context, their function may range from driving through change (an enforcement role) to facilitating change through others (a coaching role). The key message is that in the headlong rush to engineer a new approach to leadership and management in the NHS, extreme care must be taken to match the leadership and management style to particular organizational circumstances. And as circumstances change (both within and external to the organization) these should be accompanied by a re-evaluation, and where appropriate, a change in these existing approaches.

Strategic performance management

The theoretical and empirical work reported in this book holds important implications for the design of strategic approaches to performance management across the NHS (see Table 7.2). Central to this is a key strategic cultural issue pertinent to the design of per-formance management arrangements across the NHS (and within NHS organizations): the balance between checking and trusting in health care.

Whilst monitoring and measurement is important to facilitate public accountability it is evident from our empirical work that NHS trusts currently labour under a heavy burden of external checking, verification and audit. This imbalance between oversight and trust-ing is recognized in recent attempts by the UK government to loosen the corset of central control and devolve power, resources and operational freedoms to frontline organizations (manifested most clearly in the creation of foundation trusts). If greater devolution of power and responsibility is to be well placed, however, the centre needs to be confident that frontline providers can be trusted (in terms of both their competence and their motivations) to deliver the desired improvements in performance (Mannion and Davies 2002; Mannion *et al.* 2004). Striking an optimal balance between checking and trusting will therefore be crucial to the successful implementation of the latest NHS reforms.

In broad terms the benefits and drawbacks associated with checking, monitoring and measurement strategies as a lever for performance improvement are summarized in Box 7.1. A similar balance can be drawn up for policy approaches which emphasize trust (Box 7.2)

The appropriate balance between oversight and trusting will depend crucially on the nature of the process at issue. When the nature of appropriate behaviour is unambiguous and easily measured then oversight and measurement may provide useful reassurance and control for the centre. When outputs are more ambiguous

---

Box 7.1 Benefits and drawbacks of checking, monitoring and measurement

Benefits of checking, monitoring and measurement:
- Can be used to clarify an organization's objectives
- Provides information for staff to use for continuous performance improvement
- Provides data for external accountability and regulation
- Provides information for consumers to make informed choices
- Can provide a motivational force when allied to incentives

Drawbacks of checking, monitoring and measurement:
- Possibly high administrative costs
- Health care data are often inaccurate and incomplete
- Difficulties of risk adjusting for different contextual factors
- Susceptible to gaming and misrepresentation
- Is retrospective
- Often fails to capture qualitative aspects of performance
- Subject to chance variability
- Lack of fairness
- Poor reported performance may impact deleteriously on staff morale
- May crowd out some types of personal motivation

Box 7.2   Benefits and drawbacks of trusting

Benefits of trusting:
- Avoids costs associated with extensive monitoring and oversight
- In some contexts serves as a better control mechanism than either markets or hierarchies
- Can promote openness and sharing of timely and accurate information
- May enhance personal motivation because of increased levels of freedom and autonomy
- Serves as an intangible capital asset which can secure competitive advantage
- Basis for forging and maintaining partnerships, strategic alliances and professional networks
- Associated with enhanced employee satisfaction and performance
- Promotes more rapid innovation and learning in organizations
- Reduces complexity and information paralysis

Drawbacks of trusting:
- Upfront costs of building and maintaining trust can be high. However once trust has been established it can be lost or damaged very easily
- Difficult to establish who is a trustworthy agent, especially in areas where past performance might not be a good indicator of future performance
- Is a risky investment as the trustee may behave opportunistically by exploiting the vulnerability of the truster or fail to perform to expectations
- Can lead to dysfunctional 'cosy' relationships, which stifle motivation and, at the extreme, may lead to corrupt practice

---

and difficult to measure then cultural controls based on shared values and trust may be more effective (Ouchi 1980). The lesson from such an analysis is that any effective performance management system in the NHS will need to use a variety of approaches in a dynamic mix, tailored to circumstances. For example what works for surgical specialties may be inappropriate for mental health services; what works for 'excellent organizations' may be dysfunctional for 'failing' ones. Further, in an organization as complex and multi-layered as the NHS, a different mix of approaches may be appropriate for different levels of accountability (for example clinical teams reporting to a trust's directorate compared to strategic health authorities reporting to the Department of Health). What is clear is that an over-reliance on any single approach will be sure to reveal its inherent weaknesses. What is equally clear is that the strategic direction chosen for performance management will interact (sometimes facilitating, sometimes impeding) with cultural change strategies developed at the local level. The alignment of performance management strategies at all levels of the hierarchy is therefore a *sine qua non* for the growth of virtuous performance cultures in the NHS.

RESEARCH IMPLICATIONS ARISING FROM THE STUDY

This book provides evidence for the importance of organizational culture as one component of high performing health services. Yet because of the complexity of both culture and performance in modern health care systems there is still much to unravel about these important facets of organizational life. Therefore we suggest that there remains a challenging policy-focused research agenda around culture, quality and performance. Specific issues that warrant further investigation might be considered in the following areas:

- The national study of the culture/performance link in English acute trusts (reported in Chapter 5) used a cross-sectional research design. This study is valuable in that it provides a snapshot of the cultural landscape of the NHS at one point in time, and because it demonstrates some potentially important contingent relationships between culture and performance that repay more detailed study (explored in Chapters 3 and 4). Yet this study, by its very nature, will have failed to capture the dynamic nature of the culture/performance relationship. We therefore suggest that future work should build on these baseline data by adopting a longitudinal approach in which compatible data are collected at several different points in time (say every two years) from the same organizations. Such an approach may better reflect the likely lagged nature of any culture/performance link. For example our case studies showed that the current measured performance of acute trusts (e.g. the star ratings) was largely thought to be the result of historical precedent (i.e. the cultures of previous management regimes) and not necessarily the product of current practice.
- The primary care sector has until fairly recently also been largely sheltered from external performance management. At the time of the study, primary care trusts were fledgling organizations

that had barely found their feet in terms of forging effective working relationship with practices and other agencies in the health economy. Given, the nascent nature of PCTs, the new focus on measuring and managing their performance, and the considerable resources now devolved and controlled by these organizations, it would be useful to revisit the case study sites to explore how, and in what ways, culture/performance linkages evolve and transform as performance management in primary care becomes more established. The new General Medical Services contract will provide a basis and better quality data for further study of this link.

• The national survey and case studies focused on exploring the influence of senior and middle management on the cultures and performance of NHS trusts. Whilst there is some evidence to suggest that senior management cultures are the dominant influence in these areas it is also evident that cultures (and performance) are the emergent result of daily conversations and working relationships between all members of an organizational hierarchy. It would therefore be useful to explore in more depth at the micro-level how performance is accomplished *qua* culture. For example ethnographic approaches might be used to examine the distinct cultures of different clinical specialities and how these mediate, facilitate or inhibit the implementation of formal performance management arrangements. Similar approaches may also be used usefully to investigate the cultural antecedents of high quality and high safety organizations, departments, wards and clinical teams.

• Our study has highlighted a range of interventions and levers for changing the cultures of health care organizations. However few if any of these interventions have been subject to rigorous evaluation. For example research could be used assess the impact of different training and education initiatives on both cultures and performance. Such work could usefully build on the growing evidence base around interventions that lead to behavioural change in clinical practice (e.g. the EPOC Cochrane Collaboration).

• The current study demonstrated the potential for culture change to induce a range of unintended and dysfunctional consequences. It is important that any unwanted side effects of the current performance management culture are monitored, and that policies are designed to mitigate these unwanted outcomes. For example it may be worth monitoring the recruitment and retention problems of low and high performance organizations to assess whether ghettoization is taking place because of an exodus of high quality staff from low to high performing organizations. This will be particularly important as foundation trusts go live. We also heard reports of bullying, harassment and intimidation of staff to deliver the desired improvements in performance. This may therefore also be worth monitoring, particularly in zero and one star organizations where the pressures for radical change are likely to be greatest, or in three star organizations, which also evidenced significant pressures to retain their stellar status.

- Our study has highlighted the crucial role of leadership in influencing organizational cultures and performance. Given the current emphasis on replacing failing trusts' senior management teams it may be useful to explore the styles of leadership that prove successful in turning around under-performing organizations and the styles of leadership that drive high performing organizations.

- There is a real need for more and better-tested bespoke instruments for assessing cultures in NHS organizations. We used an adaptation of a US measure (the CVF), which may itself have some (national) culture specificity. It is in need of further development in the UK context. Once we have established the characteristics of desirable cultures (maybe through further intensive qualitative work) we will then be in a position to build better instruments. Given the range and diversity of issues central to culture assessment in health care, the building, testing and refining of a variety of culture instruments will be an ongoing task.

- In this book we have focused on examining the culture–performance link in English NHS trusts. There may be some merit in undertaking cross-national and inter-sectoral research in this area in order to distil the lessons from other countries and industries as they seek to implement cultural change. This may be literature-based or carried through to further empirical evaluation.

- It is clear from some of our review work (see Chapter 2) that culture may be thought of not as something internal to the organization itself, but as something co-produced by interactions with other players. Patients, carers, relatives and other health service stakeholders (such as social care workers, service commissioners or even the media) may all be important in shaping prevailing local cultures as they interact with those delivering services. Thus future studies of health service culture, especially those examining the micro-dynamics of service delivery, may need to extend their views of culture to embrace much wider groups of participants than has hitherto been the norm in culture studies.

* Although organizational culture (or community governance) through its multilateral enforcement of group norms addresses certain economic problems that cannot be handled efficiently by markets or bureaucracies, it is apparent that, like markets and bureaucracies, organizational cultures can also fail. For example organizational cultures work because they are good at enforcing group norms, and whether this is a good thing depends on how functional the norms are vis-à-vis organizational objectives. The governance limitations of organizational culture(s) are currently under-specified in the institutional economics literature and would therefore benefit from further theoretical elaboration and empirical testing.

CONCLUDING REMARKS

Organizational culture matters in organizational life, and research on organizational culture can help inform and underpin policy and management choices in health care. There is much still to learn regarding the growth and sustenance of beneficial cultures in health care and how such cultures mediate, facilitate or impede other strategies and instruments for levering performance improvement. There remains therefore a fascinating research agenda on culture/performance that sits at the intersections of policy, management, economics and a diverse array of social science. The challenge is for policy makers, funders, key stakeholders (managers, clinicians, unions, patients and carers) and researchers to work together to strengthen and broaden the evidence base that underpins thinking in this area. We offer this book as a step along the road towards that end.

APPENDIX 1: RESEARCH DESIGN AND METHODS OF DATA GATHERING AND ANALYSIS

The empirical components of the project built on, and were guided by, the review of theory and the analysis of the extant empirical evidence on culture/performance linkages. This appendix presents the logic underpinning the empirical phase of the study, and details the data gathering and analytical strategies used.

RATIONALE FOR A MULTI-METHOD APPROACH

Given the diversity of views and approaches to understanding and assessing organizational cultures we adopted a multi-method approach, integrating both qualitative and quantitative approaches in order to examine in *breadth* and *depth* any relationships between organizational culture(s) and performance as they are found in the NHS.

In attempting to capture the breadth of any inter-linkages we conducted a national quantitative survey of English acute NHS trusts, based on the competing values framework, a validated culture rating instrument. Data from this survey were then linked to a robust national performance data set (developed at the Centre for Health Economics, York). This analysis linked whole organization performance (on official measures) with self-assessed senior management team culture. We did not conduct a similar large-scale survey in primary care because the newness of primary care trusts (PCTs) reduces our ability to attribute their performance to their organizational culture. In addition, PCT-level performance data sets are far less developed than those in the acute sector.

Whilst quantitative measurements can elicit much valuable information that is amenable to rigorous statistical analysis, they are less effective in recording the dynamic processes underlying the actions recorded in the instrument. Therefore in order to provide added depth and richness to our understanding we adopted a multiple case study approach (in both acute and primary care) alongside the national survey of acute trusts to explore the internal processes and mechanisms through which 'culture' and 'performance' are mediated and accomplished within particular organizational settings. The national survey and the case studies were conducted during the same time period rather than sequentially, and both methods contribute to our overall picture of culture and its relationship to performance in the NHS.

The case studies were developed most fully in the acute care setting, where organizations are most established (in terms of formal organizational arrangements, longevity and identity). However we also explored the ideas of a culture/performance link in primary care settings. Whilst primary care organizations (PCOs) are far less developed than their acute counterparts, it is expected that they will, in time, become key drivers of health care delivery. The differences between primary care and hospital organizations meant that we were unable to adopt an identical approach in the two settings; however we used predominantly similar methods, and the project team met throughout to ensure appropriate sharing of ideas between these two aspects of the fieldwork. The scale of the project prevented us exploring the culture of other NHS organizations, such as mental health or community trusts, although clearly the issues uncovered and findings drawn may have application here also.

Case studies are typically used to explore the interplay of all organizational variables and thereby provide a more holistic or 'thick' description of a situation. In case study research generalization does not depend on conventional statistical logic. Where data are drawn from individual or multiple settings, inferences from these settings to other contexts depend on the adequacy of the theory (theoretical inference) rather than an adherence to the conventional technical rules of statistical inference. Yin (1984) describes the circumstances in which case study methods of investigation should be considered:

In general, case-studies are the preferred strategy when 'how' or 'when' questions are being posed, when the investigator has little control over events, and when the focus is on a contemporary phenomenon with some real-life context.

SECURING ROBUSTNESS IN THE CASE STUDIES

Data collection in the case studies comprised a range of sources: a culture questionnaire survey, semi-structured interviews with key managers, and a review of relevant internal and external documentation. In the analysis we triangulated evidence from each source in order to build a rich understanding of the relationship between culture and performance in each organization. The data collection from each of the sources occurred contemporaneously rather than sequentially. The output from this, in the case of the acute hospital case studies, was used to construct a holistic overview of the inter-linkages between culture and performance *within* individual organizations, with each case study possessing its own unique integrity for the purposes of inductive analysis and theoretical generalization. The case studies also formed the basis for subsequent integrative analysis and theoretical generalization *across* the acute trusts. As, at the time of the study, PCOs had less of an established identity, organizational structure or embedded organizational processes, the primary care case studies proceeded directly from data coding to an integrative analysis across sites.

It should be noted that our analysis is based on the perceptions and subjective experience of key individuals. Therefore the narrative that is presented on the linkage between culture and performance in each case study is drawn from an amalgamation of the reported subjective perceptions. In order to improve the validity of the study, where possible we cross-referenced accounts between individuals and triangulated the evidence emanating from different data sources. We attempted to reduce the potential for researcher bias by ensuring that at each stage at least two researchers analysed the data and collaborated in the development of coding categories and emergent themes. We also audited the various sources of data in order to search for negative or 'disconfirming' evidence that appeared to contradict or was inconsistent with the emerging analysis.

ASSESSING CULTURE

Culture was assessed quantitatively using the Competing Values Framework (CVF, see Chapter 5 and Cameron and Freeman 1991) which was piloted extensively before use. In the case studies, culture was also explored discursively during the interviews by asking informants to describe (and give examples of) the previous and prevailing cultures in their organization (see later sections on interviewing).

ASSESSING PERFORMANCE

Given the contested and complex nature of both performance and culture we sought to adopt flexible and adaptable definitions of both. Thus our view of performance has depended on context. In the broad quantitative analysis examining statistical associations between culture and performance we have used standardized official data sets that quantify and compare organizational performance across acute trusts. However in the qualitative case studies we applied a definition of performance that extends beyond official statistics, one that is capable of capturing qualitative dimensions of activity that defy quantification. This view also alerted us to the unintended and dysfunctional performance outcomes that are omitted from (and sometimes caused by) official lines of reporting.

DATA GATHERING FOR THE QUANTITATIVE CROSS-SECTIONAL ANALYSIS

All board-level senior managers in all English NHS acute trusts were mailed a simple questionnaire based on the competing values framework. The sampling frame was derived from a commercially available and regularly updated database that allows identification of named individuals by job specification (Binleys). Two rounds of follow-up were used to ensure a high response rate. Data on individuals' cultural perceptions were aggregated within any given trust to provide a 'trust measure' of prevalent cultural orientation. These cultural data were combined with an extensive data set on acute trust performance, which has been gathered from routinely available sources and is collated and held at the Centre for Health Economics, York (Appendix 2). Multi-variate econometric analyses using regressions, ANOVA, multi-nomial logit, ordered probit and others were used to explore the associations between measures of culture and measures of performance (explanation of the statistical approaches used is given in Appendix 2 where the models are recounted in detail).

DATA GATHERING FOR THE ACUTE HOSPITAL CASE STUDIES

Selection of the case studies

The overall aim of this arm of the project was to explore, through the use of case studies, the complex interplay between organizational culture(s) and performance in acute hospital trusts. The selection of the six trusts explored in the case studies used a three-stage process. First, we adopted a multiple case study design, which incorporated purposeful sampling of low and high performing trusts using the Department of Health star rating system. This approach we believe represents a more efficient sampling strategy than selecting a random sample of organizations. Trusts at either end of the performance spectrum are likely to offer sharper contrasts in terms of their experience and ambition for culture change and may therefore provide more valuable insights and perspectives than one based on a sample of middling performers. Moreover, given the current policy focus on 'turning around' under-performing organizations we decided to select a sample of four low performing hospital trusts (zero or one starred in the performance rating exercise) and two high performing hospital trusts (awarded three stars). To help secure confidentiality we do not identify the year of the performance rating.

Second, in order to provide useful background information, we only included trusts that had been subject to a CHI clinical governance report. Finally, we ensured that our sample comprised a mix of sizes, geographical locations and teaching/non-teaching institutions.

Of the six hospital trusts contacted, three declined to participate in the study (two one star trusts and a three star trust). We then replaced these organizations with similar trusts until we had a complement of trusts meeting the inclusion criteria.

Informant interviews

In each organization we conducted semi-structured interviews with between 8 and 11 key managers and senior clinicians. In each organization these included the chief executive and the medical director and a range of the following staff:

- Deputy chief executive
- Trust chair
- Director of finance
- Director of human resources

- Clinical directors
- Director of nursing
- Business managers

The interviews centred on a number of themes:

- The understanding of the term 'organizational culture', and the extent to which informants believed that hospitals and trusts had distinctive cultures of their own.
- Perceptions of any relationships between local cultures and possible performance, together with exemplification and explanation of these.
- A discussion of desirable and undesirable cultural traits within trusts.
- The possibility and means of managing culture (and barriers to this), including specific examples of local activities in this area.
- The means by which quality problems or performance difficulties were identified and addressed within the trust, especially the arrangements for reporting and dealing with adverse clinical events.
- The ways in which learning within and between organizations was encouraged.
- Policies and practice around developing effective strategic relationships or partnerships with external stakeholders (e.g. local PCTs, Social Services, etc.).

The above points were departures for discussions rather than a fixed schedule. Interviews were allowed to proceed as conversations, and new themes were taken up and explored as these arose.

The interviews were taped and transcribed fully prior to analysis. Transcripts were analysed using the qualitative method of content analysis with the aid of the computer analysis package Atlas ti. To increase validity of the findings the transcriptions were cross-checked against contemporaneous notes and relevant internal reports and documentation (including CHI clinical governance reports and the trusts' own clinical governance reports). Following an initial scrutiny of the transcripts several preliminary themes were identified which were discussed at a group meeting of the research team. On the basis of discussions at the meeting the transcripts were re-analysed to explore further the linkages between culture and performance in each of the cases studies. Finally, we looked for any apparent linkages between culture and performance that could be generalized across the case study sites, focusing in particular on the similarities and differences between the cultures of low performing and high performing trusts.

DATA GATHERING FOR THE PRIMARY CARE CASE STUDIES

Adopting a similar approach to that used in the acute sector arm of the project, we conducted a series of case studies in primary care trusts to explore the developing culture in PCTs and its relationship to performance. However, for a variety of reasons, we could not replicate the exact approach used in the acute trusts. First, PCTs have not yet been given star ratings, so we were unable to sample organizations using recognized published performance criteria. In addition at the time of the study there were no CHI reports on PCTs available. Second, the concept of 'organizations' in primary care is a complex and fluid one. PCTs are new organizations and most of them have more of a networked than a hierarchical structure. The constituent general practices, and sometimes teams within the practices, may have their own culture(s) and this might be very distinct from that of the PCTs. In this project, we focused principally on the culture of the PCTs, since they have similar responsibilities to acute trusts in terms of their remit to drive modernization in the NHS. However we also decided to examine the culture of the constituent practices of the PCTs when using the quantitative survey instrument, rather than the PCTs themselves, not least because of the small number of staff working in the PCTs at the time that the research was conducted. This approach allowed us to start to explore the relationship between the practices and the larger primary care organizations. As in the acute sector study, data sources used in the primary care case studies comprised semi-structured interviews, observational, documentary and survey data in order to reflect the complex and dynamic nature of culture in primary care.

SELECTION OF THE CASE STUDIES

We selected a sample of six PCTs from a purposeful sample of 12 that were already collaborating in a longitudinal programme of research into clinical governance conducted by the National Primary Care Research and Development Centre (NPCRDC) (Marshall *et al.* 2002). The sample was chosen to reflect the emphasis that we

Table A.1   Characteristics of PCT sample

Sites	Population (in 1000s)	No. of Practices	No. of GPs
A	290–330	55–65	170–210
B	200–40	27–32	110–30
C	230–70	45–55	110–30
D	130–70	23–30	80–100
E	120–60	20–7	110–30
F	90–130	15–22	50–70

knew from this study the organizations placed on cultural change in general practice, different stages of maturity (range 12–24 months since trust formation), size of the organization and geographical characteristics. Three of the PCTs approached were unable to participate in the study, either because new managers were being appointed or because they had recently undergone a time consuming review by the Commission for Health Improvement. A further three PCTs of comparable size and geographic location were then successfully recruited to take their place. The size of each of the six PCTs is shown in Table A.1 (ranges, rather than exact numbers are given to preserve anonymity); three of these had recently undergone mergers with adjacent organizations. In two of these merged PCTs (C and D) management structures were not fully in place and staff recruitment was ongoing at the time of the interviews.

THE INFORMANT INTERVIEWS

Standard letters, comprehensive research information sheets and copies of practice questionnaires were sent to the chief executives in each trust, requesting permission to interview them, together with two to three other personnel considered to have an interest in organizational culture and cultural change. Anonymity of individuals and organizations was assured. As shown below, the final sample of interviewees consisted of a range of senior and middle managers including some non-executive board members. Two of the 21 managers who agreed to take part (chief executive of Trust E and locality manager of Trust D) were subsequently unable to attend the pre-arranged interview. Interviews were carried out between April and June 2002 and all were audio-taped. The interviews lasted between

Table A.2 PCT interview sample

Sites	A	B	C	D	E	F	Totals
Chief executive	x	x				x	3
Chair (PCT)		x					1
Chair (LHG/locality)	x			x			2
Clinical governance lead	x	x	x		x	x	5
Director (LGH)	x						1
Director of service modernization				x			1
Head of service delivery						x	1
Director of nursing			x				1
Locality manager							
Community nurse man.				x			1
Non-exec. lead					x		1
Non-exec. director						x	1
Practice manager				x			1
Totals	*4*	*3*	*3*	*3*	*2*	*4*	*19*

45 and 60 minutes and were carried out by an experienced researcher at each of the PCT headquarters.

Since the aim of the study was to access the different experiences of a broad range of leaders and managers and to capture their perceptions without pre-determining their points of view, semi-structured open-ended interviews were used. The interviewer started by explaining a working definition for organization culture based on the literature and confirmed by our earlier work involving PCT managers:

> Some say that culture is about the shared attitudes, beliefs and values within an organization that impact or have the potential to impact on the way things are done in that organization – what do you think about this definition?

Once agreement about the meaning of the term had been reached, a series of themes were explored. These themes were derived from the literature and from the previous NPCRDC study on culture in PCTs (Marshall et al. 2002):

- Definitions and perceptions of PCT culture
- Definitions and perceptions of PCT performance
- The impact of collaboration between practices on culture and performance

- Possible links between culture and performance
- Strategies for cultural change to improve performance
- Facilitators and barriers to cultural change
- Autonomy and diversity in primary care

A flexible approach to the interview was taken and the interviewer followed the issues introduced or identified by the subject as being of greatest importance. The interviewer was therefore open to new or unexpected phenomenon and both the wording and sequence was adapted to different responders when necessary and the interview changed and developed as new and important themes were introduced. All interviews were taped, and the audiotapes were fully transcribed prior to analysis. For the first stage, short case summaries for each site were prepared following a format that focused on issues associated with the main interview themes and any new emerging concepts. All summaries and transcriptions were read by at least two researchers who discussed their observations before coding commenced. This was followed by a thematic content analysis in which emerging themes were allocated codes and all statements related to each theme re-examined again for further sub-themes. For greater reliability, the themes were further developed by a process of iterative review of the original transcripts and emerging ideas were shared and explored in meetings of the project team.

CONCLUDING REMARKS

The triangulation of data collection methods, data types and data sources maximized our chances of developing a comprehensive and integrated understanding of culture and the relationships between culture and performance within health care organizations. In addition, working across both secondary and primary care enabled us to explore the reach of these ideas, their wider applicability and the areas of overlap between them. Although much of the empirical work proceeded in parallel, there was considerable interplay between the different aspects of fieldwork, and the research team met frequently to share developing understandings and integrate these into ongoing data gathering.

APPENDIX 2: QUANTITATIVE MODELS AND DATA DEFINITIONS

MODEL 1: ADJUSTING FOR SENIOR MANAGEMENT ROLE

As job role may have systematic effects on the way individuals respond to the questionnaire, regressions were run on the average culture scores for each individual (group, developmental, hierarchical, rational), controlling for their job title by a set of dummy variables based on their job code. Running a fixed effect model in each case, this effectively generates an individual hospital specific effect that may be considered the 'true' hospital culture score, purged of job title effects. We therefore estimated a model of the form:

$$y_{ij} = a + x_{ij}\beta + u_i + \varepsilon_{ij}$$

where u_i is the hospital-specific residual which differs between hospitals, but for any particular hospital, its value is constant. The new 'true' hospital culture score, purged of job title effects $x_{ij}\beta$ is $(a + u_i)$, which again sums to 100 for each culture.

Fixed effects regression results of job title on culture scores

Fixed-effects (within) regression				Number of obs =			874
				Number of groups =			187
				Obs per group: min =			1
				avg =			4.7
				max =			11

R-sq: within =	0.062			0.015		0.056		0.018
between =	0.071			0.014		0.064		0.009
overall =	0.064			0.013		0.057		0.010
corr(u_i, Xb) =	0.063			0.022		0.046		−0.035
F(8,679) =	5.63			1.27		5.05		1.51
Prob > F =	0.000			0.256		0.000		0.151

Dependent variable	Clan		Developmental		Hierarchical		Rational	
	Coef.	P>|t|	Coef.	P>|t|	Coef.	P>|t|	Coef.	P>|t|
Job code 2	**−4.559**	**0.011**	−1.234	0.387	**3.391**	**0.037**	2.402	0.099
Job code 3	−2.499	0.145	0.563	0.678	1.985	0.199	−0.049	0.971
Job code 4	−2.498	0.147	−0.831	0.543	1.966	0.206	1.363	0.327
Job code 5	3.058	0.088	−2.583	0.069	−0.283	0.861	−0.192	0.895
Job code 6	**−4.401**	**0.016**	−2.605	0.073	**5.236**	**0.002**	1.770	0.232
Job code 7	**−12.581**	**0.005**	−1.077	0.762	**10.235**	**0.012**	3.423	0.344
Job code 8	7.551	0.452	−4.443	0.577	14.991	0.098	−18.099	0.026
Job code 9	**−6.112**	**0.000**	−1.536	0.248	**6.522**	**0.000**	1.126	0.406
Constant	33.849	0.000	24.161	0.000	15.741	0.000	26.249	0.000

Sigma_u	9.506		7.286		7.722		6.850	
Sigma_e	11.902		9.441		10.752		9.624	
rho (fraction of variance due to u_i)	0.389		0.373		0.340		0.336	

F test that all u_i = 0:								
F(186, 679) =	2.50		2.46		1.91		2.06	
Prob > F =	0.000		0.000		0.000		0.000	

These results suggest that job titles 2 (Director of finance), 6 (Director of HR), 7 (Director of quality) and 9 (Other) are likely to overstate hierarchical compared to clan culture. Thus we can adjust the trust culture scores as a means of removing these effects (see main text).

MODEL 2: CORRELATIONS OF TRUST CULTURE VARIABLES WITH OTHER TRUST VARIABLES

This preliminary descriptive analysis shows the correlations between various trust variables (both characteristics and performance) and trust culture variables (the scores assigned at trust-level to culture subtypes (clan, developmental, hierarchical and rational). The data are shown both weighted (for numbers of respondents in a given trust) and unweighted culture data, although the findings are substantively the same.

Correlations of culture variables with trust variables, unweighted and weighted

Trust variables	Unweighted				Weighted				n
	Clan	Develop.	Hierarch.	Rational	Clan	Develop.	Hierarch.	Rational	
Outcome variables									
Mortality index	0.089	−0.122	0.023	−0.015	0.121	−0.144	0.019	−0.023	157
Readmission rate	−0.016	0.086	0.015	−0.095	−0.025	0.053	0.072	−0.113	152
Clinical negligence	0.087	0.115	−0.153	−0.071	0.119	0.124	−0.186	−0.099	170
Complaints	**−0.372**	0.064	0.197	0.231	**−0.436**	0.042	0.257	0.283	186
Complaints resolved	0.123	0.027	−0.160	−0.017	0.128	0.046	−0.180	−0.031	186
CHI review	0.052	**0.304**	−0.264	−0.118	0.044	**0.303**	−0.287	−0.080	89
Star ratings	−0.042	0.232	−0.176	0.015	0.019	0.221	−0.221	−0.023	183
Patients trust doctor	−0.045	0.047	0.023	−0.016	−0.017	0.072	−0.030	−0.024	138
Patients trust nurses	0.078	0.027	−0.078	−0.050	0.117	0.023	−0.099	−0.084	138
Patients told doctor's name	−0.080	−0.017	0.103	0.013	−0.016	−0.025	0.060	−0.016	138
Patients single sex ward	0.149	−0.026	−0.102	−0.065	0.132	−0.064	−0.073	−0.035	138
Patients satisfied discharge procedure	0.060	−0.006	0.053	−0.143	0.138	0.006	−0.008	−0.196	138
Inpatient survey coordination of care	0.111	−0.013	−0.043	−0.095	0.165	0.025	−0.104	−0.144	170
Inpatient survey environment & facilities	0.167	−0.023	−0.091	−0.105	0.209	0.005	−0.149	−0.133	170

Inpatient survey information & education	0.056	-0.047	0.023	-0.054	0.077	-0.032	-0.004	-0.069	170
Inpatient survey physical & emotional needs	0.088	-0.011	-0.019	-0.092	0.091	0.007	-0.041	-0.090	170
Inpatient survey prompt access	0.025	0.027	-0.009	-0.055	0.067	0.042	-0.048	-0.089	170
Inpatient survey respect & dignity	0.170	0.045	-0.126	-0.143	0.214	0.066	-0.175	-0.180	170
Process variables									
ALOS	0.080	-0.062	-0.005	-0.042	0.064	-0.072	0.039	-0.056	185
Total spells	**-0.394**	0.130	0.145	0.259	**-0.472**	0.102	0.194	**0.340**	185
Total episodes	**-0.386**	0.131	0.139	0.252	**-0.466**	0.102	0.192	**0.334**	185
Total inpatient days	**-0.386**	0.097	0.167	0.256	**-0.483**	0.055	0.254	**0.340**	185
Electives	**-0.307**	0.134	0.095	0.184	**-0.336**	0.093	0.151	0.210	174
Emergencies	**-0.409**	0.126	0.158	0.271	**-0.487**	0.100	0.206	**0.357**	173
Emergency index	-0.066	-0.025	-0.014	0.136	-0.108	-0.032	-0.005	0.192	184
A&E attendances	-0.267	0.059	0.124	0.173	**-0.344**	0.046	0.183	0.231	187
Outpatients per spell	0.077	0.047	-0.034	-0.120	0.045	0.032	0.005	-0.105	186
Total first outpatient attendances	**-0.309**	0.240	0.062	0.111	**-0.385**	0.210	0.131	0.168	187
Daycases per spell	-0.095	-0.048	0.049	0.133	-0.071	-0.046	0.029	0.119	185
Delayed discharges	0.041	-0.059	0.006	0.001	0.024	-0.062	0.014	0.021	169
Occupancy	-0.074	-0.062	0.056	0.109	-0.144	-0.052	0.083	0.168	185
Vacancy rate allied health	-0.029	-0.086	0.103	0.014	-0.074	-0.113	0.163	0.049	172

Correlations of culture variables with trust variables, unweighted and weighted *continued*

Trust variables	Unweighted				Weighted				n
	Clan	*Develop.*	*Hierarch.*	*Rational*	*Clan*	*Develop.*	*Hierarch.*	*Rational*	
Vacancy rate nurses	0.051	−0.097	0.039	−0.014	−0.005	−0.103	0.071	0.042	172
Vacancy rate consultants	0.019	−0.048	0.110	−0.107	0.074	−0.074	0.102	−0.140	171
Sickness absence rate	−0.046	0.002	−0.018	0.087	−0.031	0.001	−0.052	0.104	169
Staff opinion survey	0.244	0.188	**−0.329**	−0.179	0.237	0.131	−0.262	−0.191	167
Comply with junior doctors	−0.034	0.155	−0.023	−0.093	0.034	0.154	−0.088	−0.122	170
Median wait	0.025	−0.061	−0.042	0.081	−0.005	−0.052	−0.015	0.081	185
Total inpatient wait	**−0.303**	0.144	0.074	0.191	**0.397**	0.087	0.188	0.254	186
Waiting 3 months	**−0.329**	0.176	0.075	0.192	**0.412**	0.126	0.173	0.249	186
Waiting 6 months	**−0.413**	0.115	0.151	0.290	**0.494**	0.067	0.241	**0.358**	183
Inpatient wait 18 months	−0.067	−0.050	0.089	0.047	−0.073	−0.055	0.095	0.058	180
Outpatient wait 26 weeks	0.134	−0.085	0.024	−0.128	−0.048	−0.080	0.201	−0.072	180
A&E trolley wait	0.121	−0.067	−0.014	−0.081	0.031	−0.028	0.029	−0.046	159
Waiting target	0.112	−0.065	0.009	−0.101	0.048	−0.120	0.081	−0.028	180
Cancelled ops	0.062	−0.001	−0.014	−0.072	0.044	0.006	−0.032	−0.033	170
Information governance	−0.043	0.232	−0.126	−0.042	−0.033	0.232	−0.122	−0.074	180

									N
Data quality	0.151	0.079	-0.206	-0.062	0.072	0.031	-0.148	0.031	182
Cleanliness	0.220	0.026	-0.215	-0.094	0.224	0.025	-0.194	-0.130	170
Structural variables									
Average beds	**-0.387**	0.110	0.158	0.254	**-0.466**	0.065	0.233	**0.328**	185
Free beds	**-0.338**	0.136	0.125	0.193	**-0.356**	0.094	0.167	0.214	185
Sites with more than 50 beds	**-0.306**	0.109	0.126	0.177	**-0.354**	0.083	0.199	0.192	184
WTE consultants	**-0.330**	0.126	0.176	0.139	**-0.355**	0.079	0.246	0.148	177
SHOs and HOs	**-0.317**	0.106	0.136	0.186	**-0.379**	0.039	0.254	0.213	177
WTE staff	**-0.317**	0.160	0.106	0.158	**-0.412**	0.121	0.196	0.237	186
Doctors per bed	-0.125	0.150	0.002	0.005	-0.210	0.150	0.053	0.061	157
Nurses per bed	-0.072	0.117	-0.063	0.045	-0.096	0.128	-0.060	0.054	157
Total cost	**-0.335**	0.160	0.147	0.134	**-0.410**	0.088	0.278	0.173	187
Unit cost	-0.035	0.034	0.018	-0.008	-0.083	-0.027	0.113	0.021	187
Reference cost index	0.077	-0.070	0.007	-0.043	0.061	-0.079	0.038	-0.043	185
Financial balance	0.051	0.118	-0.115	-0.067	0.014	0.100	-0.098	-0.019	180
Claiming financial support	0.113	-0.183	0.072	-0.048	0.012	-0.148	0.121	0.010	180
Retained surplus/deficit	0.096	0.087	-0.143	-0.063	0.070	0.109	-0.159	-0.039	186
Total income	-0.242	0.075	0.171	0.065	-0.273	0.013	0.275	0.065	187
Income private patients	-0.074	0.140	0.045	-0.097	-0.116	0.134	0.087	-0.079	187
Capital expenditure per bed	0.053	0.064	-0.085	-0.046	0.043	0.043	-0.040	-0.063	187
Non-salary expenditure	**-0.310**	0.125	0.158	0.122	**-0.363**	0.073	0.272	0.129	187

Correlations of culture variables with trust variables, unweighted and weighted *continued*

Trust variables	Unweighted				Weighted				n
	Clan	Develop.	Hierarch.	Rational	Clan	Develop.	Hierarch.	Rational	
Non healthcare expenditure	−0.122	0.101	−0.023	0.091	−0.146	0.009	0.059	0.131	187
Salary expenditure per WTE	−0.052	0.108	0.003	−0.045	−0.061	0.096	0.030	−0.050	186
Proportion management salaries	0.053	0.011	−0.010	−0.075	0.034	0.030	0.013	−0.095	187
Proportion consultant salaries	−0.096	0.129	−0.021	0.023	−0.143	0.131	0.012	0.045	187
Proportion nurses salaries	0.064	−0.040	−0.051	0.011	0.111	−0.060	−0.086	0.004	187
Proportion total medical salaries	−0.199	0.116	0.055	0.096	−0.252	0.097	0.104	0.135	187
Proportion non-executive salaries	0.069	0.002	−0.059	−0.032	0.031	0.017	−0.059	0.004	187
Total NHS salaries	**−0.331**	0.164	0.135	0.138	**−0.418**	0.096	0.265	0.190	187
Total salaries	**−0.336**	0.161	0.144	0.137	**−0.420**	0.093	0.274	0.185	187
Population density	−0.031	0.016	0.070	−0.053	−0.066	−0.043	0.162	−0.041	174
Market forces factor	−0.029	0.055	0.037	−0.058	−0.067	0.022	0.119	−0.060	184
Herfindahl index	−0.004	0.009	0.030	−0.040	−0.015	−0.001	0.024	−0.004	184
Heated volume per bed	0.042	0.011	−0.035	−0.030	0.055	0.011	−0.046	−0.038	184

Research revenue	−0.078	0.127	0.060	−0.092	0.111	−0.112	0.127	−0.100	184
Teaching	−0.198	0.114	0.094	0.044	0.048	−0.216	0.174	0.053	166
Students per spell	−0.091	0.033	0.088	−0.007	−0.051	−0.105	0.190	−0.009	184
SIFTR	−0.228	0.075	0.160	0.058	0.021	−0.256	0.249	0.060	187
Merged	−0.201	−0.011	0.085	0.200	−0.008	−0.189	0.060	0.208	187
Total age	**0.334**	0.181	0.062	0.209	0.153	**−0.420**	0.139	0.267	186
Casemix index	0.098	0.056	−0.042	−0.149	0.064	0.084	−0.019	−0.166	184
Population under 15	0.050	0.009	−0.024	−0.053	−0.003	0.063	−0.005	−0.081	185
Population over 60	−0.021	−0.037	−0.015	0.088	−0.025	−0.041	−0.029	0.119	185
Female population	0.028	−0.060	0.020	0.002	−0.050	0.082	−0.041	−0.015	185
Specialization index	0.240	0.098	−0.163	−0.254	0.107	0.239	−0.164	−0.269	184

Some of these variables may be collinear in a regression and may therefore not be included together. In addition, some variables (such as aspects of expenditure) may also pick up size effects and if included in the modelling may need to be adjusted in some way (for instance being logged or measured as a proportion of total expenditure).

MODEL 3: ANOVA MODELLING OF DOMINANT CULTURE AND OTHER TRUST VARIABLES

The following table shows the ANOVA results for each of the trust variables with the dominant culture variable (which is categorical). Results are shown unweighted (the weighted model was run but as this did not change results in any great way the data have not been included). The one-way ANOVA results used least squares to fit a linear model. The last column gives the significance level for the F statistic, whether the overall model is significant, and the number of observations (n).

The results are interpreted as follows (using 'complaints' as an example). The mean level of complaints for rational trusts (the omitted group) is 454. Clan culture trusts' complaints are −127 lower (significantly) at 327 (p = 0.001). Developmental culture trusts and hierarchical culture trusts have levels of complaints that appear roughly similar (insignificantly different), to those in rational culture trusts. The overall model for the regression with this variable is also significant (p = 0.000) with n = 186.

ANOVA of culture type with trust variables relative to rational culture, unweighted

Trust variables	Unweighted				
	Clan	*Develop.*	*Hierarch.*	*Rational (dropped)*	
	Coeff. $P>\lvert t\rvert$	*Coeff.* $P>\lvert t\rvert$	*Coeff.* $P>\lvert t\rvert$	*Constant* $P>\lvert t\rvert$	*n* *Prob>F*
Outcome variables	2.608	−0.381	1.778	98.000	157
Mortality index	0.231	0.902	0.680	0.000	0.579
Readmission rate	0.082	0.215	0.278	5.930	152
	0.633	0.381	0.367	0.000	0.732
Clinical	0.064	0.200	−0.200	1.000	170
negligence	0.484	0.142	0.258	0.000	0.198
Complaints	−127.27	61.17	−16.42	453.782	186
	0.001	0.267	0.817	0.000	**0.000**
Complaints	0.485	−3.950	−9.185	55.131	186
resolved	0.879	0.418	0.144	0.000	0.354
CHI review	0.300	0.446	−0.190	2.190	89
	0.173	0.161	0.681	0.000	0.314

Star ratings	0.093	0.399	0.204	1.887	183
	0.504	0.059	0.450	0.000	0.287
Patients trust	−0.174	0.695	−1.027	81.884	138
doctor	0.838	0.563	0.564	0.000	0.809
Patients trust	0.418	0.017	−1.073	78.930	138
nurses	0.608	0.988	0.530	0.000	0.812
Patients told	−0.583	0.563	−0.136	71.279	138
doctor's name	0.689	0.785	0.964	0.000	0.938
Patients single sex	2.484	3.871	−4.595	63.023	138
ward	0.480	0.438	0.534	0.000	0.654
Patients satisfied	2.045	0.055	0.867	67.419	138
discharge	0.060	0.971	0.702	0.000	0.230
procedure					
Inpatient survey	0.906	−0.576	−0.909	67.654	170
coordination of	0.221	0.597	0.517	0.000	0.284
care					
Inpatient survey	1.186	−1.074	−0.557	72.266	170
environment &	0.221	0.451	0.761	0.000	0.284
facilities					
Inpatient survey	0.249	−1.356	−1.335	68.451	170
information &	0.744	0.228	0.355	0.000	0.363
education					
Inpatient survey	0.362	−0.561	−1.256	71.051	170
physical &	0.618	0.600	0.361	0.000	0.565
emotional needs					
Inpatient survey	0.453	0.065	−1.762	79.153	170
prompt access	0.738	0.974	0.492	0.000	0.844
Inpatient survey	1.812	0.745	−1.102	81.366	170
respect &	**0.028**	0.537	0.477	0.000	0.069
dignity					

Process variables

ALOS	0.097	−0.329	0.090	3.959	185
	0.569	0.203	0.786	0.000	0.363
Total spells	−20668	5843	−7711	65857	185
	0.000	0.412	0.400	0.000	**0.000**
Total episodes	−22733	7035	−9192	72811	185
	0.000	0.378	0.371	0.000	**0.000**
Total inpatient	−73626	5086	−16754	250905	185
days	**0.000**	0.852	0.632	0.000	**0.000**
Electives	−2284	835	−1183	8348	174
	0.006	0.496	0.459	0.000	**0.007**
Emergencies	−20047	4763	−6711	59061	173
	0.000	0.482	0.446	0.000	**0.000**
Emergency index	−0.001	−0.001	−0.006	0.021	184
	0.562	0.835	0.193	0.000	0.626

Trust variables	Unweighted				
	Clan	*Develop.*	*Hierarch.*	*Rational (dropped)*	
	Coeff. P>|t|	*Coeff. P>|t|*	*Coeff. P>|t|*	*Constant P>|t|*	*n Prob>F*
A&E attendances	−15067 **0.019**	8752 0.369	10462 0.404	68008 0.000	187 **0.007**
Outpatients per spell	0.330 0.282	0.053 0.910	−0.042 0.944	3.916 0.000	186 0.685
Total first outpatient attendances	−18409 **0.000**	19005 0.016	−5136 0.611	67568 0.000	187 **0.000**
Daycases per spell	−0.013 0.384	−0.001 0.954	−0.011 0.710	0.336 0.000	185 0.826
Delayed discharges	0.142 0.796	−0.592 0.462	−0.030 0.977	4.835 0.000	169 0.814
Occupancy	−1.012 0.284	−1.740 0.226	−1.139 0.537	83.498 0.000	185 0.594
Vacancy rate allied health	−0.006 0.352	−0.005 0.640	−0.010 0.449	0.045 0.000	172 0.781
Vacancy rate nurses	0.002 0.706	−0.013 0.198	−0.001 0.926	0.036 0.000	172 0.418
Vacancy rate consultants	0.006 0.231	0.008 0.289	0.011 0.256	0.020 0.000	171 0.513
Sickness absence rate	−0.002 0.094	−0.001 0.629	−0.002 0.539	0.047 0.000	169 0.408
Staff opinion survey	0.053 **0.044**	0.019 0.624	−0.016 0.750	3.161 0.000	167 0.151
Comply with junior doctors	0.038 0.325	0.056 0.327	0.076 0.305	0.560 0.000	170 0.616
Median wait	−3.074 0.314	−6.328 0.173	−15.034 **0.012**	51.852 0.000	185 0.072
Total inpatient wait	−1892 **0.000**	530 0.465	−1395 0.136	6137 0.000	186 **0.000**
Waiting 3 months	−839 **0.000**	567 0.103	−417 0.350	2987 0.000	186 **0.000**
Waiting 6 months	−2053 **0.000**	1 0.999	−931 0.216	5383 0.000	183 **0.000**
Inpatient wait 18 months	−12.85 0.078	−13.47 0.218	−11.02 0.432	13.660 0.020	180.00 0.330
Outpatient wait 26 weeks	4.129 0.506	2.506 0.788	31.887 **0.008**	0.113 0.982	180 0.069

A&E trolley wait	−2.256	−11.899	−11.046	13.137	159
	0.775	0.294	0.447	0.033	0.683
Waiting target	1.328	−3.137	−4.237	3.045	180
	0.650	0.477	0.454	0.195	0.582
Cancelled ops	−0.003	−0.007	−0.007	0.020	170
	0.474	0.258	0.356	0.000	0.626
Information	−0.330	3.634	−1.058	21.604	180
governance	0.749	**0.020**	0.596	0.000	**0.047**
Data quality	−0.011	−0.010	−0.076	0.921	182
	0.369	0.606	**0.002**	0.000	**0.022**
Cleanliness	0.174	−0.004	−0.104	3.304	170
	0.047	0.973	0.538	0.000	0.083

Structural variables

Average beds	−260.14	31.44	−79.69	860	185.00
	0.000	0.727	0.491	0.000	**0.000**
Free beds	−41.47	25.93	−4.99	140.219	185.00
	0.000	0.119	0.815	0.000	**0.000**
Sites with more	−0.667	−0.022	0.051	2.222	184
than 50 beds	**0.000**	0.934	0.882	0.000	**0.000**
WTE consultants	−22.20	12.70	8.96	72.222	177
	0.000	0.168	0.432	0.000	**0.000**
SHOs and HOs	−20.62	13.99	9.34	79.480	177
	0.000	0.117	0.397	0.000	**0.000**
WTE staff	−802.07	327.29	−269.52	3009	186
	0.001	0.349	0.565	0.000	**0.000**
Doctors per bed	−1.498	4.265	−2.243	34.688	157
	0.399	0.094	0.525	0.000	0.103
Nurses per bed	−0.448	6.253	−4.938	118.271	157
	0.902	0.229	0.493	0.000	0.451
Total cost	−286026	165218	122194	1099299	187
	0.002	0.241	0.500	0.000	**0.000**
Unit cost	−0.009	−0.193	−0.062	1.550	187
	0.960	0.463	0.854	0.000	0.888
Reference cost	1.464	−3.262	2.396	96.731	185
index	0.533	0.362	0.602	0.000	0.515
Financial balance	0.002	0.003	0.003	−0.003	180
	0.240	0.194	0.327	0.025	0.482
Claiming	−74.95	−243.58	47.32	343.58	180
financial	0.771	0.530	0.924	0.098	0.927
support					
Retained surplus/	138.89	292.87	81.38	−691.11	186
deficit	0.562	0.423	0.863	0.000	0.868
Total income	−6145	994	9936	20874	187
	0.082	0.853	0.152	0.000	**0.043**

Trust variables	Unweighted				
	Clan	*Develop.*	*Hierarch.*	*Rational (dropped)*	
	Coeff. *P>|t|*	*Coeff.* *P>|t|*	*Coeff.* *P>|t|*	*Constant* *P>|t|*	*n* *Prob>F*
Income private	10.08	882.15	30.36	1416.182	187
patients	0.981	0.165	0.970	0.000	0.506
Capital	1430	391	654	5775	187
expenditure per bed	0.141	0.791	0.731	0.000	0.503
Non-salary	−13200000	5672595	6691206	48000000	187
expenditure	**0.006**	0.435	0.474	0.000	**0.003**
Non healthcare	−536349	−142851	−1027457	3140227	187
expenditure	0.195	0.821	0.207	0.000	0.447
Salary	570	941	1392	24144	186
expenditure per WTE	0.288	0.251	0.206	0.000	0.463
Proportion	0.000	0.001	0.006	0.042	187
management salaries	0.900	0.877	0.232	0.000	0.679
Proportion	−0.005	0.008	−0.006	0.116	187
consultant salaries	0.198	0.141	0.391	0.000	0.073
Proportion nurses	0.003	0.003	−0.009	0.374	187
salaries	0.705	0.841	0.629	0.000	0.903
Proportion total	−0.012	0.011	−0.001	0.230	187
medical salaries	**0.044**	0.220	0.962	0.000	**0.024**
Proportion non-	0.000	−0.001	−0.000	0.001	187
executive salaries	0.995	0.118	0.443	0.000	0.331
Total NHS	−17900000	10500000	4982165	69600000	187
salaries	**0.001**	0.215	0.648	0.000	**0.000**
Total salaries	−18500000	11400000	7343645	72300000	187
	0.002	0.199	0.521	0.000	**0.000**
Population	2.445	−1.024	17.571	15.629	174
density	0.520	0.862	**0.021**	0.000	0.121
Market forces	1.024	−1.020	3.018	86.598	184
factor	0.576	0.718	0.399	0.000	0.724
Herfindahl index	0.007	0.060	−0.048	0.363	184
	0.888	0.460	0.634	0.000	0.809
Heated volume	1.118	−1.784	−1.651	5.706	184
per bed	0.750	0.742	0.810	0.044	0.926

Research revenue	−0.327	0.584	0.050	2.263	184
	0.732	0.693	0.979	0.004	0.924
Teaching	−0.102	0.049	−0.007	0.189	166
	0.101	0.586	0.953	0.000	0.202
Students per spell	0.000	0.000	0.001	0.001	184
	0.914	0.299	**0.038**	0.000	0.112
SIFTR	−3468	−266	4660	11412	187
	0.173	0.945	0.352	0.000	0.245
Merged	−0.162	−0.134	−0.091	0.182	187
	0.000	0.043	0.284	0.000	**0.003**
Total age	−19387	11733	−8252	67603	186
	0.000	0.115	0.387	0.000	**0.000**
Casemix index	3.039	0.820	−0.378	92.215	184
	0.340	0.868	0.952	0.000	0.772
Population under 15	0.049	0.009	0.023	0.129	185
	0.031	0.794	0.601	0.000	0.158
Population over 60	−0.032	−0.004	−0.037	0.410	185
	0.053	0.882	0.252	0.000	0.198
Female population	0.003	−0.007	0.002	0.520	185
	0.834	0.720	0.947	0.000	0.962
Specialization index	0.254	−0.117	−0.136	0.381	184
	0.028	0.511	0.544	0.000	**0.025**

MODEL 4: EXPLAINING CULTURE TYPE BY TRUST CHARACTERISTICS (MULTI-NOMIAL LOGIT MODELLING)

In the following model we explain differences in culture type using the trust variables identified in previous analyses. We are not able to combine the separate culture scores for each trust into a single dependent variable for the model and therefore use dominant culture type in the first instance as the dependent variable. This amounts to a loss of information since trusts proportionally may belong to one culture type more than another, but not exclusively to only one. Econometrically we do not have a satisfactory way of dealing with this in a single model, since the culture scores are essentially jointly determined and constrained dependent variables.

The multi-nomial logit is the most frequently used model for nominal outcomes. A multi-nomial logit model performs maximum likelihood estimation of models with discrete dependent variables and is used when the dependent variable takes on more than two outcomes which have no natural ordering as is the case with dominant culture type. We estimate a set of coefficients $\beta^{(1)}$, $\beta^{(2)}$, $\beta^{(3)}$ and $\beta^{(4)}$ corresponding to each outcome category (for instance):

$$\Pr(y = 1) = \frac{e^{X\beta^{(1)}}}{e^{X\beta^{(1)}} + e^{X\beta^{(2)}} + e^{X\beta^{(3)}} + e^{X\beta^{(4)}}}$$

$$\Pr(y = 2) = \frac{e^{X\beta^{(2)}}}{e^{X\beta^{(1)}} + e^{X\beta^{(2)}} + e^{X\beta^{(3)}} + e^{X\beta^{(4)}}} \text{ and so on.}$$

In our case, the categories are 1, 2, 3 and 4 for each culture type clan, developmental, hierarchical and rational.

To identify the model, one of $\beta^{(1)}$, $\beta^{(2)}$, $\beta^{(3)}$ or $\beta^{(4)}$ is arbitrarily set to 0, for instance category ($y = 1$), the most frequently occurring category. Thus the remaining coefficients $\beta^{(2)}$, $\beta^{(3)}$ and $\beta^{(4)}$ measure the change relative to the ($y = 1$) group. The multi-nomial logit model can therefore be thought of as simultaneously estimating binary logits for all possible comparisons among outcome categories. Thus setting $\beta^{(1)} = 0$, the equations become (for instance):

$$\Pr(y = 1) = \frac{1}{1 + e^{X\beta^{(2)}} + e^{X\beta^{(3)}} + e^{X\beta^{(4)}}}$$

$$\Pr(y = 2) = \frac{e^{X\beta^{(2)}}}{1 + e^{X\beta^{(2)}} + e^{X\beta^{(3)}} + e^{X\beta^{(4)}}} \text{ and so on.}$$

The relative probability of ($y = 2$) to the base category ($y = 1$) is:

$$\frac{\Pr(y = 2)}{\Pr(y = 1)} = e^{X\beta^{(2)}}$$

The models are run weighted by the number of respondents per hospital. Those variables significant at the 5 percent level are highlighted, although others are significant at the 10 percent level. The model is run three times using different base categories as comparison groups in order to make all relevant contrasts across the four outcomes.

Multi-nomial logit model, weighted

Multi-nomial regression				
Number of obs =	155			
LR chi^2 (36) =	111.78			
Prob > chi^2 =	0.000			
Log likelihood =	−122.168			
Pseudo R^2 =	0.314			

Comparison group	Clan		Developmental		Hierarchical	
Dominant culture	Coefficient	P>|z|	Coefficient	P>|z|	Coefficient	P>|z|
Developmental						
Zero or one star	**−2.646**	**0.015**				
Average number of beds	**0.002**	**0.049**				
Inpatient survey respect and dignity	−0.145	0.082				
Data quality	−0.820	0.876				
Merged	2.742	0.075				
Staff opinion survey	−4.180	0.109				
Median waiting time	−0.018	0.474				
Proportion of management salaries	33.075	0.252				
Proportion of consultant salaries	**100.852**	**0.000**				
Proportion of nurses salaries	**22.297**	**0.018**				
Specialization index	−3.076	0.129				
Research revenue	**0.180**	**0.024**				
Constant	3.186	0.826				
Hierarchical						
Zero or one star	−1.728	0.212	0.917	0.578		
Average number of beds	0.003	0.070	0.001	0.655		
Inpatient survey respect and dignity	**−0.392**	**0.008**	−0.248	0.116		
Data quality	**−28.629**	**0.015**	**−27.809**	**0.024**		
Merged	**5.285**	**0.019**	2.543	0.243		
Staff opinion survey	−3.454	0.393	0.726	0.866		
Median waiting time	**−0.197**	**0.009**	**−0.179**	**0.021**		
Proportion of management salaries	**171.819**	**0.008**	**138.744**	**0.040**		
Proportion of consultant salaries	**85.368**	**0.050**	−15.484	0.735		
Proportion of nurses salaries	27.704	0.098	5.407	0.764		
Specialization index	−18.510	0.125	−15.434	0.204		
Research revenue	**0.264**	**0.036**	0.084	0.482		
Constant	48.273	0.030	45.087	0.070		
Rational						
Zero or one star	−0.237	0.681	**2.409**	**0.026**	1.491	0.275
Average number of beds	**0.003**	**0.003**	0.000	0.596	−0.000	0.891

continued

Inpatient survey respect and dignity	**−0.181**	**0.002**	−0.036	0.651	0.212	0.143
Data quality	4.902	0.213	5.722	0.305	**33.531**	**0.005**
Merged	**3.082**	**0.013**	0.340	0.766	−2.202	0.265
Staff opinion survey	**−4.449**	**0.021**	−0.269	0.911	−0.995	0.803
Median waiting time	0.005	0.735	0.023	0.357	**0.202**	**0.008**
Proportion of management salaries	30.900	0.129	−2.175	0.937	**−140.918**	**0.030**
Proportion of consultant salaries	33.883	0.065	**−66.969**	**0.008**	−51.485	0.236
Proportion of nurses salaries	5.776	0.354	−16.521	0.079	−21.928	0.198
Specialization index	0.208	0.753	3.284	0.100	18.718	0.121
Research revenue	0.097	0.072	−0.083	0.206	−0.167	0.161
Constant	14.233	0.146	11.048	0.434	−34.040	0.124

There are several tests that are commonly used in association with the multi-nomial logit (Scott Long 1997). First, we can test that all of the coefficients associated with an independent variable are simultaneously equal to zero (that is a test that a variable has no effect). We use either a likelihood-ratio test or Wald statistic to test whether the x_k variables have any effect on the dependent variable. The null hypothesis is that $H_0 : \beta_k = 0$ or that all coefficients associated with given variable(s) are zero. These statistics are distributed as chi-square and results for the likelihood-ratio test shown in the following table. All variables reject the hypothesis that they have no effect on culture types at the 10 percent significance level.

Tests of independent variables for multi-nomial logit

	LR tests		
	chi^2	df	prob > chi^2
Zero or one star	10.254	3	0.017
Average number of beds	11.137	3	0.011
Inpatient survey respect and dignity	15.643	3	0.001
Data quality	15.420	3	0.001
Merged	12.020	3	0.007
Staff opinion survey	6.518	3	0.089
Median waiting time	15.223	3	0.002
Proportion of management salaries	11.792	3	0.008
Proportion of consultant salaries	19.930	3	0.000
Proportion of nurses salaries	8.268	3	0.041
Specialization index	12.078	3	0.007
Research revenue	8.700	3	0.034

Second, we can test whether the independent variables differentiate between different pairs of outcomes. This test is commonly used to determine whether any two outcomes can be combined. Again, we can use either a likelihood-ratio test or Wald test and the null hypothesis is that all coefficients (except intercepts) associated with a given pair of outcomes are zero (or that categories can be collapsed). All pairs of outcomes are evaluated. Results for the likelihood-ratio test are shown in the following table and suggest (at the 10 percent significance level) that categories are independent and should not be collapsed.

Tests for combining dependent categories for multi-nomial logit

	LR tests		
	chi^2	df	prob > chi^2
Clan–developmental	46.322	12	0.000
Clan–hierarchical	43.438	12	0.000
Clan–rational	48.768	12	0.000
Developmental–hierarchical	25.224	12	0.014
Developmental–rational	19.624	12	0.075
Hierarchical–rational	30.284	12	0.003

Finally, we can assess the assumption of the independence of irrelevant alternatives (IIA) using a Hausman test. The multi-nomial logit assumes that the odds for any pair of outcomes are determined without reference to the other outcomes that might be available. This is known as the independence of irrelevant alternatives (IIA) property. The Hausman test is computed by estimating the full model and then a restricted model eliminating one or more outcome categories and testing the difference in the coefficients. The null hypothesis is that the difference in coefficients is not systematic. The results in the following table suggest evidence in favour of the null hypothesis in each case. Hausman and McFadden (1984) note that negative test statistics are possible and Freese and Scott Long (2000) suggest it is very common. These authors conclude that a negative result is evidence that IIA has not been violated.

Tests of IIA for multi-nomial logit

Omitted	chi²	df	prob > chi²	evidence
A	−11.679	20	–	for H_0
B	−4.008	21	–	for H_0
C	2.022	24	0.999	for H_0
D	10.070	22	0.986	for H_0

Star ratings for zero and one star trusts combined provided the best results (since zero star trusts had small numbers) whilst two and three star categories remained insignificant in all specifications. Using bed numbers controlled for size and proved significant in all specifications, hence salary expenditure variables were adjusted to reflect relative proportions of total salary expenditure (so as not to also pick up size effects). The weighting variable (number of respondents) was also tested as a potential explanatory variable since the number of respondents in a trust may be associated with the culture in terms of people being more enthusiastic or responsive to outside requests. This variable was also, however, insignificant.

MODEL 5: ORDERED PROBIT MODEL LINKING TRUST CULTURE AND TRUST STAR RATINGS

We developed an ordered probit model on the star ratings. This is derived from a model in which a latent variable y^* (performance) ranging from $-\infty$ to $+\infty$ is mapped to an observed variable y (star rating) which is thought of as providing incomplete information about the underlying y^* according to the equation:

$$y_i = m \text{ if } \tau_{m-1} \le y_i^* < \tau_m \text{ for } m = 1 \text{ to } J$$

The τs are called cutpoints. Thus for the four star ratings, zero to three, the observed y is mapped to the latent variable y^* according to the measurement model as follows:

$$y_i = \begin{cases} 0 & & \tau_0 = -\infty \le y_i^* < \tau_1 \\ 1 & & \tau_1 \le y_i^* < \tau_2 \\ 2 & \text{if} & \tau_2 \le y_i^* < \tau_3 \\ 3 & & \tau_3 \le y_i^* < \tau_4 = \infty. \end{cases}$$

Since most of the process and outcome variables were used to construct the star ratings, the only variables included are structural variables, which for the most part can be considered exogenous in the short run. In this model the culture scores are used (as opposed to culture type) in order to use the most available information on culture.

Ordered probit model of culture scores against star ratings

Ordered probit estimates			Number of obs =	159		
			LR chi^2(11) =	20.06		
			Prob > chi^2 =	0.045		
			Log likelihood =	−179.866		
			Pseudo R^2 =	0.053		

Star ratings	*Coefficient*	*Robust standard error*	*z*	*P>|z|*	*95% confidence interval*	
Culture score Clan	**−0.045**	**0.017**	**−2.690**	**0.007**	**−0.078**	**−0.012**
Culture score Hierarchical	**−0.042**	**0.014**	**−3.120**	**0.002**	**−0.069**	**−0.016**
Culture score Rational	−0.032	0.021	−1.490	0.135	−0.073	0.010
Total episodes	0.000	0.000	−1.340	0.181	0.000	0.000
Average number of beds	0.000	0.001	0.120	0.906	−0.001	0.001
Total cost	0.000	0.000	−1.590	0.112	0.000	0.000
WTE staff	**0.001**	**0.000**	**1.990**	**0.047**	**0.000**	**0.001**
Teaching	0.284	0.394	0.720	0.471	−0.488	1.057
Merged	0.091	0.360	0.250	0.800	−0.615	0.798
HRG casemix index	0.000	0.016	0.020	0.984	−0.031	0.032
MFF	0.009	0.013	0.680	0.495	−0.016	0.034
Cut 1	−4.048	2.275				
Cut 2	−2.971	2.256				
Cut 3	−1.673	2.251				

Star ratings (Probability)	Observed
0: Pr(xb+u<_cut1)	0.050
1: Pr(_cut1<xb+u<cut2)	0.208
2: Pr(_cut2<xb+u<_cut3)	0.453
3: Pr(_cut3<xb+u)	0.289

We can test using a likelihood-ratio test for the equality of coefficients across response categories, distributed as chi-square and we accept the null hypothesis (p = 0.152) that the thresholds are all about the same distance apart. We also test whether any of the categories can be combined. Again, we can use a Hausman type test by estimating the full model as well as a model with two categories combined and then test the difference in the coefficients. The null hypothesis is that the difference in coefficients is not systematic. The results suggest that categories 2 and 3 could potentially be collapsed, however this is not pursued here since the model is in essence just a verification of the relationship between culture type and star ratings and does not attempt to explain star ratings. The model was also run without the structural variables (just culture scores) and culture remained significant in explaining star ratings, though to a lesser extent. As expected, most of the structural measures included in the model are not significant in explaining any of the variation in star ratings, but it could be argued that these factors should be controlled for nonetheless to assess the 'pure' effect of culture on performance. The results seem to be consistent with the multi-nomial logit results and suggest that higher star ratings (two or three) are significantly less likely in clan and hierarchical cultures than developmental.

DATA DESCRIPTION FOR TRUST CHARACTERISTICS AND PERFORMANCE VARIABLES
(Data collated at Centre for Health Economics, University of York)

Coding for the statistical analysis had to reflect unique hospital identifiers. Trusts where mergers occurred were thus treated as, for instance, two distinct trusts merging into a trust which then becomes a third distinct unit with a new identifier code. The database covers data from 1994/95–2001/02.

CCI   (Case-mix Adjusted Unit Cost Index)

$$CCI_i = \frac{TC_i}{[(IP_i \times \underline{IC} \times HRG_i) \div (\underline{IP} \times \underline{HRG})] + [\Sigma_j OP_{ij} \times (\underline{OC_j} \div \underline{OP_j})] + [(AE_i \times \underline{AC}) \div \underline{AE}]}$$

where:

TC_i = Total cost of inpatient, outpatient and A&E care in hospital i
$\underline{IC}$ = Total cost of inpatient spells for all acute hospitals
IP_i = Number of inpatient (including day case) spells in hospital i
HRG_i = HRG case-mix index for hospital i
$\underline{IP}$ = Total number of inpatient spells for all acute hospitals
$\underline{HRG}$ = Average case-mix index for all acute hospitals

OP_{ij} = Number of first outpatient attendances across all specialties in hospital i

$\underline{OC_j}$ = Total cost of outpatient attendances for all acute hospitals in specialty j

$\underline{OP_j}$ = Number of outpatient attendances for all acute hospitals in specialty j

AE_i = Number of first A&E attendances in hospital i

$\underline{AC}$ = Total cost of A&E attendances in all acute hospitals

$\underline{AE}$ = Number of first A&E attendances in all acute hospitals

Source: DoH (Not available: 1998/99–1999/2000)

2CCI Case-mix Costliness Adjusted Unit Cost Index)

A unit cost measure which takes account of additional adjusters over and above the CCI of hospital output and factor prices.

Source: DoH (not available: 1998/99–1999/2000)

3CCI Case-mix Costliness & Configuration Adjusted Unit Cost Index)

A unit cost measure which takes account of additional adjusters over and above the 2CCI of structural and environmental factors.

Source: DoH (not available: 1998/99–1999/2000)

RCI (Reference Cost Index)

A weighted average of Healthcare Resource Group (HRG) costs in a trust relative to the national average. The RCI gives a single figure for each NHS trust that compares the actual cost for its case-mix with the same case-mix calculated using national average costs.

Source: DoH (not available: 1994/95–1997/98)

RCI+ (Reference Cost Index (plus))

The RCI+ indicator was an estimate of the RCI adjusted for a series of legitimate cost drivers. Data from routine trust returns was incorporated to give the best estimate of the RCI extended to cover expenditure on inpatients (including daycases), outpatients, daycare and A&E in all general and acute and maternity specialities.

Source: DoH (not available: 1994/95–1998/99)

TUC2000   (Trust Unit Cost 2000)

An efficiency indicator which is a percentage ratio of the actual RCI+ divided by the expected RCI+.

Source: DoH (not available: 1994/95–1999/00 (outside of database)

UNIT COSTS   (Total costs divided by weighted activity)

$$C_{it} = \frac{TC_{it}}{[(IP_{it} \times \underline{IC_t} \times HRG_{it}) \div (\underline{IP_t} \times \underline{HRG_t})] + [(OP_{it} \times \underline{OC_t}) \div \underline{OP_t}] + [(AE_{it} \times \underline{AC_t}) \div \underline{AE_t}]}$$

where:

C_{it} = Unit cost for hospital i in period t

TC_{it} = Total cost incurred by hospital i in period t

IP_{it} = Number of inpatient spells in hospital i in period t

$\underline{IC_t}$ = Total costs incurred for inpatient spells for all acute hospitals in period t

HRG_{it} = HRG case mix index for hospital i in period t

$\underline{IP_t}$ = Total number of inpatient spells for all acute hospitals in period t

$\underline{HRG_t}$ = Average HRG case mix index for all spells treated for all acute hospitals in period t

OP_{it} = Total first outpatient attendances in hospital i in period t

$\underline{OC_t}$ = Total cost of outpatient attendances for all acute hospitals in period t

$\underline{OP_t}$ = Total first outpatient attendances for all acute hospitals in period t

AE_{it} = Total A&E attendances in hospital i in period t

$\underline{AC_t}$ = Total cost of A&E attendances in all acute hospitals in period t

$\underline{AE_t}$ = Total A&E attendances in all acute hospitals in period t

Hospitals where geriatrics and psychiatry constituted more than 50 percent of admissions were also excluded from the hospital level analyses because of an inability to adequately capture the output of such institutions. Previous work suggests that HRGs do not perform well for these specialties (Söderlund *et al.* 1996), where diagnosis is typically a poor predictor of resource use. However mental health activity in mainly acute hospitals is included for completeness, despite some problems with HRGs in this category.

Source: Derived from variables described

TC   (Total cost)

These costs are total expenditure divided by the GDP deflator with 1995 as the base year and include all activity, capital charges, labour, teaching and research costs.

Source: CIPFA

GDP DEFLATOR   (Deflator for NHS costs)

1995 used as the base year.

Source: HM Treasury

CHNGUCOST   (Change in unit costs from period t–1 to t)
    Source: Derived from unit cost variable described (not available: 1994/95–1995/96)

IP   (Total inpatient spells

Inpatient activity data includes daycases, where these admissions simply have a 0 length of stay.
        Source: CIPFA; Hospital Episode Statistics (HES)

IC   (Total inpatient cost)

Source: CIPFA

OP   (Total first outpatient attendances)

Source: CIPFA

OC   (Total outpatient cost)

Source: CIPFA

AE   (Total accident and emergency (A&E) attendances)
Source: CIPFA

AC   (Total accident and emergency (A&E) cost)
Source: CIPFA

EMERG ADMISN   (Number of emergency admissions)
Source: Hospital Episode Statistics (HES)

EMERG_INDEX   (Standardized index of unexpected emergency admissions/total emergencies)

This variable reflects additional costs associated with coping with unpredictable demand. The variable is calculated as the 12-month sum of the absolute value of residuals from a simple model of emergency admissions standardized to give an index with a national average of one. A single regression was run for the whole sample using provider specific dummies with each month's emergency demand set as a function of the previous month's demand plus a monthly dummy.

Source: DoH (not available: 1998/99–1999/2000)

HRG   (HRG case-mix index)

In order to estimate a case mix index for a hospital, all cases were allocated to a healthcare resource group (HRG) category (Benton *et al.* 1998), and a weight representing the expected cost of that category attached accordingly. The average cost weight for all spells treated over a year formed the scalar case mix index for that hospital. The national average case weight was set to equal 100, and case mix indices above 100 thus represent hospitals that have treated a more complex than average mix of cases.

Source: DoH (not available: 1998/99–1999/2000
(assumed constant from 1997/98)

IT_INDEX   (Information Theory specialization index)

Single specialty hospitals are likely to draw patients from further afield and have greater short-term variation in demand for services because of the lack of cross-specialty compensation effects. Economies of specialization might occur where relatively under-utilized, specialized fixed resources are centralized in one institution, rather than spread over many. This can be examined through the inclusion of an Information Theory Index which calculates the degree to which the proportions of different case-types (HRGs) in a hospital differ from the national average proportion of case-types. The formula used for derivation of the Information Theory Index as calculated by Farley (Farley 1989; Farley and Hogan 1990) is given below:

$$ITI_h = \Sigma_i \, P_{ih} \log \left(P_{ih}/\pi_i \right)$$

where ITI_h is the case mix specialization index for hospital h, P_{ih} is the proportion of cases in hospital h that fall into HRG i, and π_i is the proportion of all hospitals' caseload constituted by HRG i. An increased IT index indicates a relatively more specialized hospital (one with a narrower scope of activities) which one would expect to be of higher cost. General hospitals typically have an IT index of between 0.2 and 0.5, whereas this may increase up to 2.5 in a highly specialized, single discipline hospital.

The literature suggests that non-price competitive pressures to introduce technology changes have driven increased specialization (Luft *et al.* 1986; Farley and Hogan 1990). Evidence suggesting better quality of care when hospitals treat higher volumes of certain medical conditions and procedures also tends to favour some specialization (Flood *et al.* 1984; Hughes *et al.* 1987; Luft *et al.* 1987).

Despite the fact that both the case-mix index HRG and IT_INDEX use HRGs in their construction, the specialization index and the HRG case-mix index are fundamentally different. The former simply captures the range of different types of cases treated, whereas the latter captures the average resource intensity of cases.

PROP15   (Proportion of patients under 15 years of age)

This variable measures whether social expectations may force trusts to expend more resources on younger patients, diagnosis and other factors being equal (Söderlund *et al.* 1995).

Source: Hospital Episode Statistics (HES)

PROP60   (Proportion of patients over 60 years of age)

Elderly patients are likely to have more complex care needs, and these may not be captured entirely by HRGs, which have only limited age sensitivity.

Source: Hospital Episode Statistics (HES)

PROPFEM   (Proportion of female patients)

This variable captures any gender-specific differences in resource need, other case-mix factors being equal.

Source: Hospital Episode Statistics (HES)

IPDAYS_SPELL   (Inpatient days per spell (proxy for average length of stay)
Source: Hospital Episode Statistics (HES)

LOS   (Actual divided by expected length of stay (according to national average)

Above unity represents longer than expected length of stay.
Source: Hospital Episode Statistics (HES)

EMERG_SPELL   (Proportion of spells that involve an emergency admission)

Large fluctuations in levels of emergency admissions imply that more fixed capacity has to be retained for a given average level of activity and, consequently, costs should increase. This variable measures whether, diagnostic case-mix and other factors being equal, emergencies will be more costly than elective admissions because of the implied threat of serious adverse outcome.
Source: DoH; Hospital Episode Statistics (HES)

DAYCASE_SPELL   (Proportion of daycases per spell)
Source: Hospital Episode Statistics (HES) (not available: 1994/95)

TRANSIN_SPELL   (Proportion of spells that involve a transfer in from another hospital)

Transfers into a hospital are likely to represent difficult or problem cases referred from less capable institutions and are thus likely to be cost-increasing.
Source: DoH (not available: 1998/99–1999/2000)

TRANSOUT_SPELL   (Proportion of spells that end in a transfer to another hospital)

It is assumed that transfers from a hospital represent an inability to meet the treatment needs of a given case. Transfers out of a hospital are likely to represent incomplete treatment of cases and are thus likely to be cost-decreasing.
Source: DoH (not available: 1998/99–1999/2000)

FCE_SPELL   (Proportion of spells involving a transfer in from another specialty)

Measurement of the volume of inpatient care performed by NHS acute hospitals has been the finished consultant episode (FCE). During a single hospital admission, however, multiple FCEs might occur as a result of transfers within or between specialties. The inpatient spell, or set of episodes constituting a single admission, thus serves as a slightly higher level of aggregation of inpatient activity. Although the FCE has been extensively criticized, it is argued that spells also fail to fully capture total inpatient activity. Spells requiring inter-specialty transfers are likely to be more complex and costly than those which can be fully treated within a specialty. This variable captures the additional effect of inter-specialty transfers over and above the average multiple FCE.

Source: DoH (not available: 1998/99–1999/2000)

EP_SPELL   (Average NHS inpatient episodes per NHS inpatient spell)

Although treatment spells (whole admissions) is the measure of volume of inpatient activity for trusts, the episodes variable incorporates the fact that volume of inpatient activity is represented by two variables (the spell and the episode). It is argued that the true unitary measure of volume of inpatient activity probably lies somewhere between the spell and the episode.

Source: Hospital Episode Statistics (HES)

OP_SPELL   (Non-primary outpatient attendances per inpatient spell)

The basic unit of outpatient activity is assumed to consist of first rather than follow-up outpatient attendances, based on information which suggests that many follow-up outpatient attendances occur because of a failure to complete treatment during the first attendance. Since follow-up attendances may, however, in some instances constitute genuine additional health care output, this variable has been included as a regressor.

Source: Hospital Episode Statistics (HES)

AVBEDS   (Average available beds)

While hospital managers do have some control over the size and capacity of their institution, it is expected that there will be some inability to radically alter capacity in the short run. This variable reflects the average daily number of available beds, for wards open overnight (for 24 hours).

Source: DoH

FREEBEDS   (Average number of free available beds)

This is derived as the average number of available beds minus (the average number of available beds times the occupancy rate).

Source: Derived from avbeds and occupancy (not available: 1994/95–1995/96

OCCUPANCY   (Average occupancy rate)

This reflects the average daily number of occupied beds divided by the average daily number of available beds (avbeds), for wards open overnight (i.e. 24 hours). It is for general and acute.

Source: DoH (not available: 1994/95–1995/96)

STUDENT_SPELL   (Medical student whole time teaching equivalents per inpatient spell)

Student whole-time equivalents (WTEs) are used as an indicator of the amount of teaching done by a hospital. The data relates to two NHS Executive Surveys in 1992/3 and 1997/8. Figures for intervening years were calculated by means of a weighted moving average.

Source: NHS Executive; DoH (not available: 1998/99–1999/2000 (assumed constant from 1997/98))

TEACHING   (Trust teaching status)

A dummy variable taking the value 1 if a trust has teaching status according to the Department of Health trust clustering group 210.

Source: DoH

RESEARCH   (Percentage of total revenue spent on research)

The data relates to a survey conducted by the NHS Executive in 1994 (Söderlund *et al.* 1996).

Source: NHS Executive; DoH (not available: 1998/99–1999/2000 (assumed constant from 1997/98))

SURPLUS_1   (Retained financial surplus or deficit)

The variable is lagged.

Source: CIPFA (not available: 1994/95)

TARGETPC   (Percentage reduction required in unit costs from efficiency target)

Source: Health Authority PEIs in Appendix 2 for 1996/97 and 1997/98; NHS Executive for 1999/2000 onwards (not available: 1994/95–1995/96; 1998/99)

MFF   (Market forces factor)

Market prices for inputs including land, buildings and labour differ between trusts because of their geographic location. This variable is a weighted average of staff, land, buildings and London weighting factors which represent an unavoidable influence on hospital costs. Component price indices are weighted according to their proportional contribution nationally in constructing the index.

Source: DoH

HEATBED   (Heated volume per bed in cubic metres)

This variable captures inefficiencies in how hospital buildings are used to create treatment capacity (represented by beds). A large amount of heated volume per bed is assumed to represent less efficient use of capital and thus cost increasing.

Source: DoH (not available: 1998/99–1999/2000)

SALARY_WTE   (Salary expenditure per whole-time equivalent staff)

Salary expenditure is deflated by GDP deflator.

Source: CIPFA

CAPITAL_BED   (Capital expenditure per bed)

Capital expenditure reflects depreciation and amortization charges, deflated by the GDP deflator.

Source: CIPFA

SITES50B   (Number of sites with more than 50 beds)

Trusts that are located on a number of sites, rather than concentrated in one location, are likely to suffer from duplication of certain capital and staff inputs, as well as incurring communication and management difficulties, thus increasing costs. The number of major sites with more than 50 beds was chosen to exclude sites that were simply isolated accommodation, chronic care or outpatient facilities.

Source: DoH (not available: 1998/99–1999/2000)

WAIT3MN   (Number of patients waiting for three months for inpatient treatment)

Hospital inpatient waiting list statistics data obtained from the KH07 quarterly returns of patients waiting to be admitted to NHS hospitals either as a day case or ordinary admission. Data was taken as at the fourth quarter of each year.

Source: DoH (*The Green Book*)

WAIT6MN   (Number of patients waiting for six months for inpatient treatment)

Hospital inpatient waiting list statistics data obtained from the KH07 quarterly returns of patients waiting to be admitted to NHS hospitals either as a day case or ordinary admission. Data was taken as at the fourth quarter of each year.

Source: DoH (*The Green Book*)

MEDIANWAIT   (Median waiting time for an inpatient admission)

Source: DoH; Hospital Episode Statistics (HES) (not available: 1994/95)

TOTWAIT **(Total number waiting for inpatient treatment)**
Source: DoH (*The Green Book*)

READMISN **(Readmission rate)**

The variable measures emergency readmissions that occur within 28 days of being discharged per 100,000 admissions. Adjusted for age, but not gender or socio-economic status.
Source: DoH Clinical Indicators (not available: 1994/95)

DIS_HIP **(Patients who return to usual place of residence within 28 days following a hip fracture)**

This variable reflects the fact that restoring function and well-being of hip fracture patients would represent a successful health outcome in rehabilitating such patients. Eight weeks is considered an appropriate period of rehabilitation. Whilst the proportion of those who return to pre-hip fracture level of accommodation will depend partly on the availability of support at home or the quality of community services, a change in the category of accommodation may suggest an important change in health status. Measured as percentage of continuous stays of patients with hip fracture. Adjusted for age, but not gender or socio-economic status.
Source: DoH Clinical Indicators (not available: 1994/95)

DIS_STROKE **(Patients who return to usual place of residence within 56 days following a stroke)**

This variable reflects the fact that restoring function and well-being of stroke patients would represent a successful health outcome in rehabilitating such patients. Four weeks is considered an appropriate period of rehabilitation. Whilst the proportion of those who return to pre-stroke level of accommodation will depend partly on the availability of support at home or the quality of community services, a change in the category of accommodation may suggest an important change in health status. Measured as percentage of continuous stays of patients with stroke. Adjusted for age, but not gender or socio-economic status.
Source: DoH Clinical Indicators (not available: 1994/95)

DEATH_HEART   (Deaths within 30 days of emergency admission of patients with heart attack)

For patients over 50 years of age, measured per 100,000 stays of patients with heart attack (as an emergency admission). Adjusted for age, but not gender or socio-economic status. Thirty-day death rates for acute myocardial infarction have been shown to be good predictors of seven day and one year death rates in US data (McClellan and Staiger 1999).

Source: DoH Clinical Indicators (not available: 1994/95)

DEATH_HIP   (Deaths within 30 days of emergency admission of patients with hip fracture)

For patients over 65 years of age, measured per 100,000 stays of patients with hip fracture (as an emergency admission). Adjusted for age, but not gender or socio-economic status.

Source: DoH Clinical Indicators (not available: 1994/95)

DEATH_NE_SURG   (Deaths within 30 days following a non-emergency admission for surgery)

Measured per 100,000 stays of patients following non-emergency surgery. Adjusted for age, but not gender or socio-economic status.

Source: DoH Clinical Indicators (not available: 1994/95)

DEATH_E_SURG   (Deaths within 30 days following an emergency admission for surgery)

Measured per 100,000 stays of patients following emergency surgery. The risk of dying after surgery will depend in part on whether the surgery was pre-planned or an emergency response to an acute condition and are therefore separate variables (emergency and non-emergency admissions). Adjusted for age, but not gender or socio-economic status.

Source: DoH Clinical Indicators (not available: 1994/95)

MORTALITY   (Dummy variable based on mortality index)

Dummy takes a value of 1 if mortality is less than national average standardized to equal 100. Based on four-year average standardized mortality index adjusted for age, sex, primary diagnosis, length of stay and type of admission.

Source: Dr Foster *Your Hospital Guide* (not available: 1994/95–1998/99)

DOCTORS_BED (Dummy variable based on number of doctors per 100 hospital beds)

Takes value of 1 if staff numbers are higher than national average. Average for England: 35.

Source: Dr Foster *Your Hospital Guide* (not available: 1994/95–1998/99)

NURSE_BED (Dummy variable based on number of nurses per 100 hospital beds)

Takes value of 1 if staff numbers are higher than national average. Average for England: 119.

Source: Dr Foster *Your Hospital Guide* (not available: 1994/95–1998/99)

TRUST_DOCTOR (Percentage of patients that have trust and confidence in their doctor)

During 1999 the Department of Health surveyed 112,000 patients who had been seen with heart disease. An average of 435 patients per NHS trust responded to the questionnaire which reflects satisfaction with overall treatment received by heart patients. Average in England: 83%. Best performing trust in England: 94%.

Source: Dr Foster *Your Hospital Guide* (not available: 1994/95–1998/99)

TRUST_NURSE (Percentage of patients that have trust and confidence in all the nurses)

During 1999 the Department of Health surveyed 112,000 patients who had been seen with heart disease. An average of 435 patients per NHS trust responded to the questionnaire which reflects satisfaction with overall treatment received by heart patients. Average in England: 79%. Best performing trust in England: 88%.

Source: Dr Foster *Your Hospital Guide* (not available: 1994/95–1998/99)

DOCTOR_NAME   (Percentage of patients that were told the name of the doctor in overall charge of their care)

During 1999 the Department of Health surveyed 112,000 patients who had been seen with heart disease. An average of 435 patients per NHS trust responded to the questionnaire which reflects satisfaction with overall treatment received by heart patients. Average in England: 73%. Best performing trust in England: 89%.

Source: Dr Foster *Your Hospital Guide* (not available: 1994/95–1998/99)

SINGLE_SEX   (Percentage of patients that stayed in a single-sex ward or room throughout their stay)

During 1999 the Department of Health surveyed 112,000 patients who had been seen with heart disease. An average of 435 patients per NHS trust responded to the questionnaire which reflects satisfaction with overall treatment received by heart patients. Average in England: 65%. Best performing trust in England: 96%.

Source: Dr Foster *Your Hospital Guide* (not available: 1994/95–1998/99)

DISCHARGE   (Percentage of patients that felt staff took their family or home situation into account when planning their discharge)

During 1999 the Department of Health surveyed 112,000 patients who had been seen with heart disease. An average of 435 patients per NHS trust responded to the questionnaire which reflects satisfaction with overall treatment received by heart patients. Average in England: 69%. Best performing trust in England: 82%.

Source: Dr Foster *Your Hospital Guide* (not available: 1994/95–1998/99)

REFERENCES

Allaire, Y. and Firsirotu, M. (1984) Theories of organizational culture, *Organization Studies*, 5: 193–226.

Alpander, G. (1990) Relationship between commitment to hospital goals and job satisfaction: a case study of a nursing department, *Health Care Management Review*, 15: 51–62.

Altman, D.G. and Bland, J.M. (1995) Absence of evidence is not evidence of absence, *British Medical Journal*, 311: 485.

Alvesson, M. (1995) *Cultural Perspectives on Organisations*. Cambridge: Cambridge University Press.

Alvesson, M. and Willmott, H. (2002) Identity regulation as organizational control: producing the appropriate individual, *Journal of Management Studies*, 39(5): 619–44.

Argote, L. (1989) Agreement about norms and work-unit effectiveness: evidence from the field, *Basic and Applied Social Psychology*, 10(2): 131–40.

Ashkanasy, N.M. and Jackson, C.R.A. (2001) Organizational culture and climate, in N. Anderson, D.S. Ones, H.K. Sinangil and C. Viswesvaran (eds) *Handbook of Industrial, Work and Organizational Psychology, Volume 2: Organizational Psychology*. Thousand Oaks: Sage Publications.

Bass, B. (1985) *Leadership and Performance beyond Expectations*. New York: Free Press.

Bate, P. (1999) *Strategies for Cultural Change*. Oxford: Butterworth-Heinemann.

Becker, G.S. (1976) *The Economic Approach to Human Behaviour*. Chicago: University of Chicago Press.

Beer, M., Eisenstat, R.A. and Spector, B. (1990) Why changes programs don't produce change, *Harvard Business Review*, 68(Nov.–Dec.): 158–66.

Bennis, W. and Nanus, B. (1985) *Leaders: The Strategies for Taking Charge*. New York: Harper & Row.

Benton, P.L., Antony, P. Evans, H. *et al.* (1998) The development of healthcare resources groups, version 3, *Journal of Public Health Medicine*, 20: 351–8.

Bourn, M. and Ezzamel, M. (1986) Organisational culture in hospitals in the NHS, *Financial Accountability and Management*, 2(3): 203–25.

Bower, P., Campbell, S., Bojke, C. and Sibbald, B. (2003) Team structure, team climate and the quality of care in primary care: an observational study, *Quality and Safety in Health Care*, Aug. (12): 273–9.

Bowles, S. (1998) Endogenous preferences: the cultural consequences of markets and other economic institutions, *Journal of Economic Literature*, 36: 75–111.

Brennan, T., Leape, L. and Laird, N. (1991) Incidence of adverse events and negligence in hospitalized patients: results of the Harvard Medical Practice Study I, *New England Journal of Medicine*, 324: 370–6.

Broadbent, J., Laughlin, R. and Shearn, D. (1992) Recent financial and administrative changes in general practice: an unhealthy intrusion into medical autonomy, *Financial Accountability*, 8: 129–48.

Brooks, I. and Brown, R. (2002) The role of ritualistic ceremonial in removing barriers between subculture in the National Health Service, *Journal of Advanced Nursing*, 38: 341–52.

Brown, A. (1995) *Organizational Culture*. London: Pitman.

Bryman, A. (1996) Leadership in organizations, in S. Clegg, C. Hardy and W. Nord (eds) *Handbook of Organization Studies*. London: Sage.

Cameron, K. and Freeman, S. (1991) Culture, congruence, strength and type: relationship to effectiveness, *Research in Organizational Change and Development*, 5: 23–58.

Carrillo, J.D. and Gromb, D. (1999) On the strength of corporate cultures, *European Economic Review*, 43: 1021–37.

Carroll, J., Rudolph, J. and Hatakenaka, S. (2002) Lessons learned from non-medical industries: root cause analysis as culture change at a chemical plant, *Quality and Safety in Health Care*, 11: 266–9.

Checkland, P. (1994) Systems theory and management thinking, *American Behavioral Scientist*, 38(1): 75–91.

Child, J. and Faulkner, D. (1998) *Strategies of Co-operation: Managing Alliances, Networks, and Joint Ventures*. Oxford: Oxford University Press.

Clegg, S. (1990) *Modern Organisations: Organisation Studies in the Postmodern World*. London: Sage.

Coeling, H. and Simms, L. (1993) Facilitating innovation at the nursing unit level through cultural assessment, Part 1: how to keep management ideas from falling on deaf ears, *Journal of Nursing Administration*, 23: 46–53.

Coleman, J.S. (1990) *Foundations of Social Theory*. Cambridge: Belknap Press of Harvard University Press.

Conger, J. (1989) *The Charismatic Leader: Behind the Mystique of Exceptional Leadership*. San Francisco: Jossey-Bass.

Cooke, R.A. and Lafferty, J.C. (1987) *Organisational Culture Inventory (OCI)*. Plymouth, MI: Human Synergistics.

Cyert, R. and March, J. (1963) *A Behavioural Theory of the Firm.* Englewood Cliffs, NJ: Prentice Hall.

Davies, H.T.O. (1999) Falling public trust in health services: implications for accountability, *Journal of Health Services Research and Policy*, 4(4): 193–4.

Davies, H.T.O. (2002) Understanding organizational culture in reforming the National Health Service, *Journal of the Royal Society of Medicine*, 95: 140–2.

Davies, H.T.O. and Mannion, R. (1999) The rise of oversight and the decline of mutuality in the NHS, *Public Money and Management*, 19(2): 55–9.

Davies, H.T.O. and Mannion, R. (2000) Clinical governance: striking a balance between checking and trusting, in P.C. Smith (ed.) *Reforming Health Care Markets: An Economic Perspective.* Buckingham: Open University Press.

Davies, H.T.O. and Nutley, S. (2000) Developing learning organisations in the NHS, *British Medical Journal*, 320: 998–1001.

Davies, H.T.O., Nutley, S.M. and Mannion, R. (2000) Organisational culture and health care quality, *Quality in Health Care*, 9: 111–19.

Deal, T.E. and Kennedy, A.A. (1982) *Corporate Cultures.* Reading, MA: Addison-Wesley.

Deal, T.E. and Kennedy, A.A. (1992) *Corporate Cultures: The Rites and Rituals of Corporate Life.* London: Penguin.

Deci, E.L. and Ryan, R. (1987) The support of autonomy and the control of behaviour, *Journal of Personality and Social Psychology*, 53: 1024–37.

Degeling, P., Kennedy, J., Hill, M., Carnegie, M. and Holt, J. (1998) Do professional subcultures set the limits of hospital reform? *Clinician in Management*, 7: 89–98.

Degeling, P., Maxwell, S., Kennedy, J. and Coyle, B. (2003) Medicine, management and modernisation a 'danse macabre'? *British Medical Journal*, 326: 649–52.

Denison, D.R. (1990) *Corporate Culture and Organizational Effectiveness.* Chichester: John Wiley & Sons.

Denison, D.R. (1996) What *is* the difference between organizational culture and organizational climate? A native's point of view on a decade of paradigm wars, *Academy of Management Review*, 21: 619–54.

Department of Health (1997) *The New NHS: Modern, Dependable.* London: The Stationery Office.

Department of Health (1998) *A First Class Service: Quality in the New NHS.* London: Department of Health.

Department of Health (2000a) *The NHS Plan. A Plan for Investment. A Plan for Reform.* London: Department of Health.

Department of Health (2000b) *An Organisation with a Memory: Report of an Expert Group on Learning from Adverse Events in the NHS Chaired by the Chief Medical Officer.* London: Department of Health.

Department of Health (2001a) *Learning from Bristol: the Department of Health's Response to the Report of the Public Inquiry into Children's Heart*

Surgery at the Bristol Royal Infirmary 1984–1995. London: Department of Health.

Department of Health (2001b) *Shifting the Balance of Power: Securing Delivery*. London: Department of Health.

Department of Health (2001c) *Shifting the Balance of Power: The Next Steps*. London: Department of Health.

Department of Health (2001d) *Building a Safer NHS for Patients*. London: Department of Health.

Department of Health (2002a) *Delivering the NHS Plan, Next Steps on Investment, Next Steps on Reform*. London: Department of Health.

Department of Health (2002b) *NHS Foundation Trusts: Eligibility Criteria and Timetable*. London: Department of Health.

Department of Health (2003) *Raising Standards: Improving Performance in the NHS*. London: The Stationery Office.

DHSS (1984) *Health Services Management: Implementation of the NHS Management Inquiry*. London: DHSS.

Donaldson, L.J. (1998) Clinical governance: a statutory duty for quality improvement [editorial], *Journal of Epidemiology and Community Health*, 52(2): 73–4.

Douglas, M. (1985) Introduction, in J.L. Gross and S. Rayner (eds) *Measuring Culture: A Paradigm for the Analysis of Social Organization*. New York: Columbia University Press.

Farley, D.E. (1989) Measuring casemix specialization and the concentration of diagnoses in hospitals using information theory, *Journal of Health Economics*, 8: 185–207.

Farley, D.E. and Hogan, C. (1990) Case-mix specialization in the market for hospital services, *Health Services Research*, 25: 757–83.

Fey, C.F. and Beamish, P.W. (2001) Organizational climate similarity and performance: international joint ventures in Russia, *Organization Studies*, 22: 853–82.

Firth-Cozens, J., Redfern, N. and Moss, F. (2002) *Confronting Errors in Patient Care: Report on Focus Groups*, Working paper. Birmingham: Faculty of Public Health, University of Birmingham.

Flood, A.B., Scott, W.R. and Ewy, W. (1984) Does practice make perfect? Parts I and II, *Medical Care*, 22(2): 98–124.

Foucault, M. (1972) *Power/Knowledge*. New York: Free Press.

Freese, J. and Scott Long, J. (2000) Tests for the multinomial logit model, *Stata Technical Bulletin*, 58: 19–25.

Fuchs, V.R. (2000) The future of health economics, *Journal of Health Economics*, 19: 141–57.

Fukuyama, F. (1995) *Trust: The Social Virtues and the Creation of Prosperity*. New York: Free Press.

Fulop, N., Protopsaltis, G., Hutchings, A. *et al.* (2002) Process and impact of mergers of NHS trusts: multicentre case study and management cost analysis, *British Medical Journal*, 323: 246–9.

Gergen, K. (1992) Organisation theory in a postmodern era, in M. Reed and

M. Hough (eds) *Rethinking Organisation Theory and Analysis*. London: Sage.

Gerowitz, M.B. (1998) Do TQM interventions change management culture? Findings and implications, *Quality Management in Health Care*, 6(3): 1–11.

Gerowitz, M.B., Lemieux-Charles, L., Heginbothan, C. and Johnson, B. (1996) Top management culture and performance in Canadian, UK and US hospitals, *Health Services Management Research*, 9: 69–78.

Gillies, R., Shortell, S. and Radamaker, A. (1992) Culture survey. Berkeley, CA: Health Policy and Management, School of Public Health.

Goddard, M. and Mannion, R. (1998) From competition to co-operation: new economic relationships in the National Health Service, *Health Economics*, 7: 105–19.

Goddard, M., Mannion, R. and Smith, P. (1999) Assessing the performance of NHS hospital trusts: the role of 'hard' and 'soft' information, *Health Policy*, 48: 119–34.

Goddard, M., Mannion, R. and Smith, P. (2000) Enhancing performance in health care: a theoretical perspective on agency and the role of information, *Health Economics*, 9: 95–107.

Gordon, G.G. and Di Tomaso, N. (1992) Predicting corporate performance from organizational culture, *Journal of Management Studies*, 29(6): 783–98.

Gosbee, J. (2002) Human factors engineering and patient safety, *Quality and Safety in Health Care*, 11: 352–4.

Grol, R. (1997) Beliefs and evidence in changing clinical practice, *British Medical Journal*, 315: 418–21.

Gudeman, S. (1986) *Knowledge as Culture*. London: Routledge and Kegan Paul.

Handy, C. (1988) *Understanding Organisations*. Middlesex: Penguin.

Harris, L.C. and Ogbonna, E. (1998) Employee reactions to organizational culture change efforts, *Human Resource Management Journal*, 8: 78–92.

Harris, L.C. and Ogbonna, E. (2002) The unintended consequences of culture interventions: a study of unexpected outcomes, *British Journal of Management*, 13: 31–49.

Harrison, J. and Nutley, S.M. (1996) Professions and management in the public sector: the experience of local government and the NHS in Britain, in J. Leopold, I. Glover and M. Hughes (eds) *Beyond Reason? The National Health Service and the Limits of Management*. Aldershot: Avebury.

Harrison, S., Hunter, D.J., Marnoch, G. and Pollit, C. (1989) General management and medical autonomy in the National Health Service, *Health Services Management Research*, 2(1): 38–46.

Harrison, S., Hunter, D.J., Marnoch, G. and Pollit, C. (1992) *Just Managing: Power and Culture in the National Health Service*. London: Macmillan.

Hausman, J.A. and McFadden, D. (1984) Specification tests for the multinomial logit model, *Econometrica*, 52: 1219–40.

Hawkins, P. (1997) Organizational culture: sailing between evangelism and complexity, *Human Relations*, 50: 417–40.

Hermalin, B.E. (2000) *Economics and Corporate Culture*. Berkeley, CA: Department of Economics, University of California.

Higgins, J. (2001) The listening blank, *Health Service Journal*, 111 (95772): 22–5.

Hodgson, G.M. (1996) Corporate Culture and the Nature of the Firm, in J. Groenewegen (ed.) *Transaction Cost Economics and Beyond*. Boston: Kluwer Academic Press.

Hofstede, G. (1980) *Culture's Consequences: International Differences in Work-Related Values*. Beverly Hills, CA: Sage.

Hofstede, G. (1994) *Cultures and Organisations: Software of the Mind*. London: HarperCollins.

Hughes, R.G., Hunt, S.S. and Maerki, S.C. (1987) Effects of surgeon volume and hospital volume on quality of care in hospitals, *Medical Care*, 25(6): 489–503.

Iles, V. and Sutherland, K. (2001) *Organisational Change. A Review for Health Care Managers, Professionals and Researchers*. London: NCCSDO.

Institute of Medicine (1999) *To Err is Human: Building a Safer Health System*. Washington, DC: National Academy Press.

Institute of Medicine (2000) *Crossing the Quality Chasm: A New Health System for the 21st Century Committee on Quality of Health Care in America*. Washington, DC: Institute of Medicine.

Jackson, S. (1997) Does organizational culture affect out-patient DNA rates? *Health Manpower Management*, 23(6).

Jones, C. and Dewing, I. (1997) The attitudes of NHS clinicians and medical managers towards changes in accounting controls, *Financial Accountability and Management*, 13: 261–80.

Kasper, W. and Streit, M. (1998) *Institutional Economics: Social Order and Public Policy*. Aldershot: Edward Elgar.

Katzner, D.W. (2002) What are the questions? *Journal of Post Keynesian Economics*, 25(1): 51–68.

Kennedy, I. (2001) *Learning from Bristol: Public Inquiry into Children's Heart Surgery at the Bristol Royal Infirmary 1984–1995*. London: The Stationery Office.

Kilmann, R. (1984) *Beyond the Quick Fix: Managing Five Tracks to Organizational Success*. San Francisco: Jossey-Bass.

Kohn, L., Corrigon, J. and Donaldson, M. (eds) (2000) *To Err is Human: Building a Safer Health System*. Washington, DC: National Academy Press.

Kotter, J. (1990) *A Force for Change: How Leadership Differs from Management*. New York: Free Press.

Kotter, J. and Heskett, J. (1992) *Corporate Culture and Performance*. New York: Macmillan.

Krackhardt, D. and Stern, R. (1988) Informal networks and organizational crisis: an experimental simulation, *Social Psychology Quarterly*, 51: 123–40.

Kralewski, J., Wingert, T. and Barbouche, M. (1996) Assessing the culture of medical group practices, *Medical Care*, 34: 377–88.

Kreps, D.M. (1990) Corporate culture and economic theory, in J.E. Alt and K.A. Shepsle (eds) *Perspectives on Positive Political Economy*. Cambridge: Cambridge University Press.

Langfield-Smith, K. (1995) Organisational culture and control, in A. Berry, J. Broadbent and D. Otley (eds) *Management Control: Theories, Issues and Practices*. London: Macmillan.

Le Grand, J., Mays, N. and Mulligan, J. (eds) (1998) *Learning from the NHS Internal Market: A Review of the Evidence*. London: King's Fund.

Legge, K. (1994) Managing culture: fact or fiction, in K. Sisson (ed.) *Personnel Management: a Comprehensive Guide to Theory and Practice in Britain*. Oxford: Blackwell.

Lindbeck, A. (1995) Welfare state disincentives with endogenous habits and norms, *Scandinavian Journal of Economics*, 47: 477–94.

Locock, L. (1999) *Leadership, Change and Primary Care Groups*. London: Office of Health Economics.

Luft, H.S., Robinson, J.C., Garnick, D.W., Maerki, S.C. and McPhee, S.J. (1986) The role of specialized clinical services in competition among hospitals, *Inquiry*, 23: 83–94.

Luft, H.S., Hunt, S.S. and Maerki, S.C. (1987) The volume–outcome relationship: practice makes perfect or selective referral patterns? *Health Service Research*, 22(2): 157–82.

Lundberg, C. (1985) On the feasibility of cultural intervention, in P. Frost, L. Moore, M. Louis, C. Lundberg and J. Martin (eds) *Reframing Organizational Culture*. Newbury Park, CA: Sage.

Machlup, F. (1981) *Knowledge: Its Creation, Distribution and Economic Significance*. Princeton: Princeton University Press.

Mannion, R. and Davies, H.T.O. (2002) A principal-agent perspective on clinical governance, in D. Kernick (ed.) *Getting Health Economics into Practice*. Oxford: Radcliffe Medical Press.

Mannion, R. and Goddard, M. (2001) Impact of published clinical outcomes data: case study in NHS hospital trusts, *British Medical Journal*, 323: 260–3.

Mannion, R. and Goddard, M. (2002) Performance measurement and improvement in health care, *Applied Health Economics and Health Policy*, 1(1): 13–23.

Mannion, R. and Small, N. (1999) Postmodern health economics, *Health Care Analysis*, 7: 255–72.

Mannion, R., Davies, H.T.O. and Marshall, M.N. (2003) *Impact of 'Star' Performance Ratings on English Acute Trusts: Secondary Analysis of Case-study Evidence*. London: Commission of Health Improvement.

Mannion, R., Goddard, M., Kuhn, M. and Bate, A. (2004) *Earned Autonomy in the NHS* (a report for the Department of Health) York: Centre for Health Economics, University of York.

Marshall, M., Sheaff, R., Campbell, S. *et al.* (2002) A qualitative study of cultural changes in primary care organisations needed to implement clinical governance, *British Journal of General Practice*, 52: 641–5.

Martin, J. (1992) *Culture in Organizations: Three Perspectives*. New York: Oxford University Press.

Martin, J. and Seihl, C. (1983) Organizational culture and counterculture: an uneasy symbiosis, *Organizational Dynamics*, 12: 52–64.

Mayhew, A. (1994) Culture, in G.M. Hodgson *et al.* (eds) *The Elgar Companion to Institutional and Evolutionary Economics*. Aldershot: Edward Elgar.

McClellan, M. and Staiger, D. (1999) *The Quality of Health Care Providers*, Working Paper 7327. Cambridge, MA: National Bureau of Economic Research.

Miles, R. and Snow, C. (1978) *Organizational Strategy, Structure and Process*. New York: McGraw-Hill.

Mintzberg, H. (1983) *Power In and Around Organisations*. Englewood Cliffs, NJ: Prentice-Hall.

Morgan, G. (1986) *Images of Organization*. London: Sage.

NHS Executive (1998) *The New NHS: Modern and Dependable. A National Framework for Assessing Performance*. Leeds: NHS Executive.

Nieva, V. (2002) *United States/United Kingdom Patient Safety Research Methodology Workshop: Measuring Patient Safety Culture*. London: The Agency for Healthcare Research and Quality/The Patient Safety Research Programme.

Nieva, V. and Sorra, J. (2003) Safety culture assessment: a tool for improving patient safety in health care organisations, *Quality and Safety in Healthcare*, 12(supp. 2): 17–23.

North, D.C. (1990) *Institutions, Institutional Change and Economic Performance*. Cambridge: Cambridge University Press.

Nystrom, P.C. (1993) Organizational cultures, strategies, and commitments in health care organizations, *Health Care Management Review*, 18(1): 43–9.

Ormrod, S. (2003) Organisational culture in health service policy and research 'third way' political fad or policy development, *Policy and Politics*, 31: 227–37.

Ott, J.S. (1989) *The Organizational Culture Perspective*. Chicago: Dorsey.

Ouchi, W.G. (1979) A conceptual framework for the design of organisational control systems, *Management Science*, 25: 833–49.

Ouchi, W.G. (1980) Markets, bureaucracies, and clans, *Administrative Sciences Quarterly*, 25: 129–41.

Ouchi, W.G. (1981) *Theory Z: How American Business Can Meet the Japanese Challenge*. Reading, MA: Addison-Wesley.

Ouchi, W. and Wilkins, A. (1985) Organizational culture, *Annual Review of Sociology*, 11: 457–83.

Pascale, R. Millemann, M. and Gioja, L. (1997) Changing the way we change, *Harvard Business Review*, Nov.–Dec.

Payne, R.L. (2000) Climate and culture: how close can they get? In N.M. Ashkanasy, C.P.M. Wilderom and M.F. Peterson (eds) *Handbook of Organizational Culture and Climate*. Thousand Oaks, CA: Sage Publications.

Peters, T. and Waterman, R. (1982) *In Search of Excellence: Lessons from America's Best Run Companies*. New York: Harper and Rowe.

Pettigrew, A. (1979) On studying organizational culture, *Administrative Science Quarterly*, 24: 570–81.

Pidgeon, N. (1997) The limits to safety? Culture, politics, learning and man-made disasters, *Journal of Contingencies and Crisis Management*, 5(1): 1–14.

Pizzi, L., Goldfarb, N. and Nash, D. (2003) Promoting a culture of safety, in R. Wachter and M. McDonald (eds). *Making Health Care Safer: A Critical Analysis of Patient Safety Practices*. Report prepared for Agency for Healthcare Research and Quality. San Francisco: Stanford University Evidence-based Practice Center, University of California at San Francisco.

Reason, J. (1997) *Managing the Risks of Organisational Accidents*. Aldershot: Ashgate.

Rizzo, J.A., Gilman, M.P. and Mersmann, C.A. (1994) Facilitating care delivery: redesign using measures of unit culture and work characteristics, *Journal of Nursing Administration*, 24(5): 32–7.

Roethlisberger, F. and Dixon, W. (1939) *Management and the Worker: An Account of a Research Program Conducted by the Western Electric Company*. Cambridge, MA: Harvard University Press.

Saffold, G.S. (1988) Culture traits, strength, and organizational performance: moving beyond strong culture, *Academy of Management Review*, 13: 546–58.

Sashkin, M. (1988) The visionary leader, in J. Conger and R. Kanungo (eds) *Charismatic Leadership: The Elusive Factor in Organizational Effectiveness*. San Francisco: Jossey-Bass.

Scally, G. and Donaldson, L.J. (1998) Clinical governance and the drive for quality improvement in the new NHS in England, *British Medical Journal*, 317: 61–5.

Schein, E. (1985a) How culture forms, develops and changes, in R. Kilmann, M. Saxton, R. Serpa and associates (eds) *Gaining Control of the Corporate Culture*. San Francisco: Josse- Bass.

Schein, E.H. (1985b) *Organisational Culture and Leadership*. San Francisco: Jossey-Bass.

Schein, E.H. (1990) Organisational culture, *American Psychologist*, 45(2): 109–19.

Schein, E.H. (2000) Sense and nonsense about culture and climate, in

N.M. Ashkanasy, C.P.M. Wilderom and M.F. Peterson (eds) *Handbook of Organizational Culture and Climate*. Thousand Oaks, CA: Sage Publications.

Schneider, B. (1990) *Organizational Culture and Climate*. San Francisco: Jossey-Bass.

Schneider, B. and Reichers, A. (1983) On the etiology of climates, *Personnel Psychology*, 36: 19–39.

Scott Long, J. (1997) *Regression Models for Categorical and Limited Dependent Variables*. London: Sage Publications.

Scott, J.T., Mannion, R., Davies, H.T.O. and Marshall, M. (2001) *Organisational Culture and Performance in the NHS: A Review of the Theory, Instruments and Evidence*. York: Centre for Health Economics.

Scott, J., Mannion, R., Davies, H.T.O. and Marshall M (2003a) *Health Care Performance and Organisational Culture*. Oxford: Radcliffe Medical Press.

Scott, J.T., Mannion, R., Davies, H.T.O. and Marshall, M. (2003b) Does organisational culture influence health care performance? A review of the evidence, *Journal of Health Services Research and Policy*, 8(2): 105–17.

Scott, J.T., Mannion, R., Davies, H.T.O and Marshall, M. (2003c) Implementing culture change in health care: theory and practice, *International Journal of Health Care Quality*, 15(2): 111–18.

Scott, J., Mannion, R., Davies, H.T.O. and Marshall, M. (2003d) The quantitative measurement of organisational culture in health care: a review of the available instruments, *Health Services Research*, 38: 923–45.

Seel, R. (2000) New insights on organisational change, *Organisations & People*, 7: 2–9.

Selznick, P. (1957) *Leadership in Administration: A Sociological Interpretation*. New York: Harper & Row.

Senge, P. (1985) *The Fifth Discipline: The Art and Practice of the Learning Organization*. New York: Doubleday Currency.

Shortell, S.M., Waters, T.M., Clarke, K.B. and Budetti, P.P. (1998) Physicians as double agents: maintaining trust in an era of multiple accountabilities, *Journal of the American Medical Association*, 280 1102–8.

Shortell, S., Jones, R., Rademaker, A. *et al.* (2000) Assessing the impact of total quality management and organizational culture on multiple outcomes of care for coronary artery bypass graft surgery patients, *Medical Care*, 38(2): 201–17.

Shortell, S.M., Lazzali, J.L., Burns, L.R. *et al.* (2001) Implementing evidence-based medicine. The role of market pressures, compensation incentives, and culture in physician organizations, *Medical Care*, 39(7): I-62–I-78.

Singer, S., Gaba, J., Geppert, A. *et al.* (2003) The culture of safety: results of an organization-wide survey in 15 California hospitals, *Quality and Safety in Health Care*, 12: 112–18.

Smelser, N.J. (1992) Culture: coherent or incoherent, in R. Munch and N.J. Smelser (eds) *Theory of Culture*. Berkley: University of California Press.

Smircich, L. (1983) Concepts of culture and organization analysis, *Administrative Science Quarterly*, 28: 339–58.

Smircich, L. and Morgan, G. (1982) Leadership: The management of meaning, *Journal of Applied Behavioral Science*, 18(3): 257–73.

Smith, P. (1995a) On the unintended consequences of publishing performance data in the public sector, *International Journal of Public Administration*, 18: 277–310.

Smith, P.C. (1995b) Outcome-related performance indicators and organizational control in the public sector, in J. Holloway, J. Lewis and G. Mallory (eds) *Performance Measurement and Evaluation*. London: Sage.

Smith, P.C. (ed.) (2000) *Reforming Markets in Health Care – An Economic Perspective*. Buckingham: Open University Press.

Smith, P.C. (ed.) (2002) *Measuring Up: Improving Health System Performance in OECD Countries*. Paris: OECD.

Smith, P., Mannion, R. and Goddard, M. (2003) Performance management in health care: information, incentives and culture. HM Treasury Public Services Productivity Discussion Papers, HM Treasury, London.

Söderlund, N., Milne, R., Gray, A. and Raferty, J. (1995) Differences in hospital casemix, and the relationship between casemix and hospital costs, *Journal of Public Health and Medicine*, 17: 25–32.

Söderlund, N., Gray, A. Milne, R. and Raftery, J. (1996) Case mix measurement in English hospitals: an evaluation of five methods for predicting resource use, *Journal of Health Services Research and Policy*, 1: 10–19.

Sutherland, K. and Dawson, S. (1998) Power and quality improvement in the new NHS: the roles of doctors and managers, *Quality in Health Care*, 7(Suppl.): S16–S23.

Throsby, D. (2001) *Economics and Culture*. Cambridge: Cambridge University Press.

Vincent, D., Taylor-Adams, S., Chapman, E.J. *et al.* (2000) How to investigate and analyse clinical incidents: Clinical Risk Unit and Association of Litigation and Risk Management protocol, *British Medical Journal*, 320: 777–81.

Walshe, K. and Higgins, J. (2002) The use and impact of inquiries in the NHS, *British Medical Journal*, 325: 895–900.

Weick, K., Sutcliffe, K. and Obstfeld, D. (1999) Organizing for high reliability: processes of collective mindfulness, *Research in Organizational Behaviour*, 21: 81–123.

West, M. (2002) How can good performance among doctors be maintained? *British Medical Journal*, 325: 669–70.

Wilderom, C.P.M., Glunk, U. and Maslowski, R. (2000) Organizational culture as a predictor or organizational performance, in N.M. Ashkanasy, C.P.M. Wilderom and M.F. Peterson (eds) *Handbook of Organizational Culture and Climate*. Thousand Oaks, CA: Sage Publications.

Williams, A., Dobson, P. and Peters, C. (1996) *Changing Culture: New Organisational Approaches*. London: Institute of Personnel and Development.

Williams, R. (1983) *Keywords: A Vocabulary of Culture and Society*. New York: Oxford University Press.
Willmott, H. (1993) Strength is ignorance; slavery is freedom: managing culture in modern organizations, *Journal of Management Studies*, 30(4): 515–52.
Wilson, D. (1992) *A Strategy of Change: Concepts and Controversies in the Management of Change*. London: Routledge.
Wilson, R.M., Runciman, W.R., Gibberd, R.W. *et al.* (1995) The quality in Australian health care study, *Medical Journal of Australia*, 163: 458–71.
Yin, R. (1984) *Case Study Research: Design and Methods*. Beverly Hills, CA: Sage.
Zaleznik, A. (1977) Managers and leaders: are they different? *Harvard Business Review*, 55: 67–78.
Zimmerman, J., Shortell, S.M., Rousseau, D.M. *et al.* (1993) Improving intensive care: observations based on organizational case studies in nine intensive care units. A prospective, multicentre study, *Critical Care Medicine* 21(10): 1443–51.
Zimmerman, J., Shortell, S.M., Rousseau, D.M. *et al.* (1994) Intensive care at two teaching hospitals: an organizational case study, *American Journal of Critical Care*, 3(2): 129–38.

INDEX

REASONABLE RATIONING
INTERNATIONAL EXPERIENCE OF PRIORITY SETTING IN HEALTH CARE

Chris Ham and Glenn Robert (Eds)

Reasonable Rationing is must reading for those interested in how to connect theory about fair rationing processes to country-level practices. The five case studies reveal a deep tension between political pressures to accommodate interest group demands and ethically motivated efforts to improve both information and institutional procedures for setting fair limits to care. The authors frame the issues insightfully.

Professor Norman Daniels, Harvard School of Public Health

- How are different countries setting priorities for health care?
- What role does information and evidence on cost and effectiveness play?
- How are institutions contributing to priority setting?
- What are the lessons for policy makers?

Priority setting in health care is an issue of increasing importance. Choices about the use of health care budgets are inescapable and difficult. A number of countries have sought to strengthen their approach to priority setting by drawing on research-based evidence on the cost and effectiveness of different treatments. This book brings together leading experts in the field to summarize and analyse the experience of priority setting in five countries: Canada, The Netherlands, New Zealand, Norway and the United Kingdom. Drawing on literature from a range of disciplines, it makes a significant contribution to the debate on the role of information and institutions in priority setting.

Reasonable Rationing has been written with a broad readership in mind. It will be of interest to policy makers, health care professionals and health service managers, as well as students of health and social policy at advanced undergraduate and postgraduate levels.

Contents

192pp   0 335 21185 2 (Paperback)   0 335 21186 0 (Hardback)

THE EUROPEAN PATIENT OF THE FUTURE

Angela Coulter and Helen Magee (Eds)

Health care is changing fast and patients' experiences and expectations are also changing. Developments in information technology and biotechnology are already having a profound influence on the way health services are delivered and the organization of health care is under reform in most countries. Patients no longer see themselves as passive recipients of care: increasingly they expect to be involved in all decisions that affect them.

This book reports the results of a major study carried out in eight different European countries to look at health policy dilemmas through the eyes of the patient. Drawing on literature reviews, focus groups and a survey of 1000 people in each of the eight countries, the book addresses the following questions:

- Why might the patients of the future be different?
- What will patients and citizens expect from health systems?
- Will the public be willing to pay more for better health care?
- What kind of value trade-offs are people prepared to make, for example between prompt access and continuity of care, or between choice and equity?
- How will patients access information, advice and treatment?
- How should policy-makers and providers react to patients' desire for greater autonomy?
- How can public confidence in health systems be maintained in the future?

The European Patient of the Future is a clear, jargon-free text which will be a key resource for all health service professionals, health policy analysts and patient advocates.

Contents

Series editor's introduction – Introduction – Health services in the different countries – Germany – Italy – Poland – Slovenia – Spain – Sweden – Switzerland – United Kingdom – Communication, information, involvement and choice – Key issues for European patients – Appendix – Index.

224pp   0 335 21187 9 (Paperback)   0 335 21188 7 (Hardback)

REGULATING HEALTHCARE
A PRESCRIPTION FOR IMPROVEMENT?

Kieran Walshe

Healthcare organizations in the UK and the USA face a growing tide of regulation, accreditation, inspection and external review, aimed at improving their performance. In the USA, over three decades of healthcare regulation by state and federal government and by non-governmental agencies have created a complex, costly and overlapping network of oversight arrangements for healthcare organizations. In the UK's government run National Health Service, regulation is central to current health policy, with the creation of a host of new national agencies and inspectorates tasked with overseeing the performance of NHS hospitals and other organizations.

But does regulation work? This book:

- Explores the development and use of healthcare regulation in both countries, comparing and contrasting their experience and drawing on regulatory research in other industries and settings.
- Offers a structured approach to analysing what regulators do and how they work.
- Develops principles for effective regulation, aimed at maximizing the benefits of regulatory interventions and minimizing their costs.

Regulating Healthcare will be read by those with an interest or involvement in health policy and management, including policy makers, healthcare managers, health professionals and students. It is particularly suitable for use on postgraduate health and health related programmes.

Contents

c. 224pp   0 335 21022 8 (Paperback)   0 335 21023 6 (Hardback)

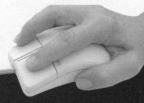
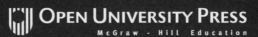